Caroline Joy Co, PT, DPT,

Current Evidence Based Protocols on the use of Therapeutic Modalities

Ultrasound, Iontophoresis,
Low Level Laser Therapy, Electrical Stimulation and
Spinal Decompression

Current Evidence Based Protocols on the use of Therapeutic Modalities

ISBN:1452821860
EAN-13: 9781452821863
Printed in the United States of America

Disclaimer:

This book is intended for informational and educational purposes only. It is not meant to provide any medical advice. Many of the product names referred to herein are trademarks or registered trademarks of their respective owners. Care has been taken to confirm the accuracy of the information presented and to describe generally accepted practices. However, the authors, editors, and publisher are not responsible for errors or omissions or for any consequences from application of the information in this book and make no warranty, expressed or implied, with respect to the currency, completeness, or accuracy of the contents of the publication. Application of this information in a particular situation remains the professional responsibility of the practitioner.

Rehabsurge, Inc.'s mission is to support healthcare and education professionals to continue their educational and professional development. Rehabsurge is committed to identifying, promoting, and implementing innovative continuing education activities that can increase and impart professional knowledge and skills through books, audiobooks, or digital e-books based on sound scientific and clinically derived research. The first Rehabsurge continuing education book was published in July 2009.

As a sponsor of Continuing Education (CE) seminars and workshops, we enable professionals to enhance their skills, pursue professional interests, and redefine their specialties within their respective disciplines while earning CEUs, CE credits, or Contact Hours. Offerings include CE books, audiobooks, and digital e-books, all of which are focused on the latest treatment and assessment approaches and include discussions of alternative and state-of-the art therapies.

Rehabsurge exists to provide the latest treatment and assessment approaches to the practicing clinician. The basic proposition of our business is simple, solid, and timeless. When we bring the latest knowledge and skill to our clients, we successfully nurture and protect our brand. That is the key to fulfilling our ultimate obligation to provide consistently attractive books, audiobooks, and digital e-books.

For permissions and additional information contact us:
Rehabsurge, Inc.
PO Box 287 Baldwin, NY 11510.
Phone: +1 (516) 515-1267
Email: ceu@rehabsurge.com

Current research in your fingertips
REHAB SURGE
Use evidence in your practice now!

DISABILITY POLICY:

Rehabsurge seeks to ensure that all students have access to its activities. To that end, it is committed to providing support services and assistance for equal access for learners with disabilities. Rehabsurge has a firm commitment to meeting the guidelines of the Americans with Disabilities Act and Section 504 of the Rehabilitation Act of 1973. Rehabsurge will provide support services and assistance for students with disabilities, including reasonable accommodations, modifications, and appropriate services to all learners with documented disabilities.

About the Author
Caroline Joy Co, PT, DPT, CHT, CSFA, is a licensed physical therapist and certified hand therapist whose clinical experience includes acute, subacute, home health, and outpatient settings. Her background includes Community-Based Therapy that is designed to help people with disabilities access therapy in their communities. She is the President and CEO of PTSponsor.com, an online resource for U.S. hospitals and clinics that seek to sponsor and hire foreign-trained rehabilitation therapists. She specializes in hand therapy through an integrated approach that includes education, counsel, and exercise. She is also certified in functional assessment for work hardening and work conditioning. Co is also the President of Rehabsurge, a continuing education company and a contracting agency. Her past affiliations include Long Beach Medical Center, Horizon Health and Subacute Center, and Grandell Therapy and Nursing Center.
Co was a professional speaker for Summit Professional Education, Cross Country Education and Dogwood Institute. She received her transitional doctorate from A.T. Still University and her BS in Physical Therapy from University of the Philippines College of Allied Medical Professions. She is licensed in California, Nevada, and New York.

Full Disclosure
To comply with professional boards/associations standards, all planners, speakers, and reviewers involved in the development of continuing education content are required to disclose their relevant financial relationships. An individual has a relevant financial relationship if he or she has a financial relationship in any amount occurring in the last 12 months, with any commercial interest whose products or services are discussed in their presentation content over which the individual has control. Relevant financial relationships must be disclosed to the audience.

As part of its accreditation with boards/associations, Rehabsurge, Inc. is required to "resolve" any reported conflicts of interest prior to the educational activity. The presentation will be scientifically balanced and free of commercial bias or influence.

To comply with professional boards/associations standards:

I declare that neither I nor my family has any financial relationship in any amount occurring in the last 12 months, with a commercial interest whose products or services are discussed in my presentation. Additionally all planners involved do not have any financial relationship.

Caroline Joy Co, PT, DPT, CHT, CSFA

Course Description

This publication explores the effectiveness of several therapeutic modalities in the treatment of neurological and musculoskeletal disabilities and the challenges faced by health practitioners in selecting the most appropriate treatments. Numerous guidelines recommend therapeutic modalities for the management of musculoskeletal conditions; however, recommendations are lacking concerning the specific adjunct modalities to employ. This review will also discuss current evidence-based clinical practice guidelines that have been developed in the treatment of neurological and musculoskeletal conditions.

Clinicians use a variety of modalities to reduce pain, improve mobility, and treat neuromusculoskeletal injuries and disabilities. Examples of therapeutic modalities include hot packs, cold packs, whirlpools, TENS (Transcutaneous Electrical Nerve Stimulation), ultrasound, traction, electrical stimulation, and joint and spine mobilization/manipulation, all of which can help strengthen, relax, and heal muscles, as well as expedite recovery in the orthopedic setting.

Course Objectives

1. Understand how ultrasound benefits fracture healing.

2. Identify the mechanisms of action of iontophoresis, low-level laser therapy, electrical stimulation, and spinal decompression therapy.

3. Choose the best modalities for osteoarthritis and rheumatoid arthritis.

4. Prescribe the best treatment protocol for knee pain, neck pain, and shoulder pain based on evidence-based guidelines.

5. Differentiate between high-intensity and low-intensity ultrasound.

TABLE OF CONTENTS/COURSE OUTLINE

CHAPTER 6 **COMMON MEDICATIONS**

Clinicians use a variety of modalities to reduce pain, improve mobility, and treat neuromusculoskeletal injuries and disabilities. Examples of therapeutic modalities include hot packs, cold packs, whirlpools, TENS (Transcutaneous Electrical Nerve Stimulation), ultrasound, traction, electrical stimulation, and joint and spine mobilization/manipulation, all of which can help strengthen, relax, and heal muscles, as well as expedite recovery in the orthopedic setting. Numerous guidelines recommend therapy for the management of musculoskeletal conditions; however, recommendations are lacking concerning the specific adjunct modalities to employ. Any prescription should include the diagnosis; type, frequency, and duration of the prescribed therapy; therapeutic goals; and safety precautions.

This review will explore the effectiveness of several therapeutic modalities in the treatment of neurological and musculoskeletal disabilities and the challenges faced by the health practitioner in selecting the most appropriate treatments. It will also describe evidence-based clinical practice guidelines for several musculoskeletal disorders.

Evidence-Based Clinical Practice Guidelines

Evidence-based clinical practice guidelines are defined by the Institute of Medicine as recommended interventions for specific clinical conditions that are based on scientific literature (Scalzitti 2001). A guideline can only be as good as the evidence on which it is based. As new evidence is identified, certain recommendations may no longer be appropriate. Therefore, revisions are necessary to ensure that a guideline is based on the best current evidence (Scalzitti 2001).

The appearance of terms such as systematic within practice guidelines does not ensure that the guidelines were developed using a structured review format. Methods to review the literature vary. Therefore, the minimal criteria for any practice guideline should include explicit statements that explain the process of creating the recommendation and gauging the evidence. The absence of such description should cause users to question the validity of the guideline.

Evidence-based clinical practice guidelines are designed to assist both practitioner and patient in making decisions about appropriate health care for specific clinical circumstances, yet the responsibility remains with the clinician to combine this evidence with clinical expertise and patient values in managing individual patients and achieving optimal outcomes.

Evidence-based clinical practice guidelines are one of four types of guidelines. The simplest type is based on expert consensus. Since these guidelines are based on the opinions of experts, and not on evidence, a lower level of applicability is usually associated with them. Expert-based guidelines are limited in that they may reflect only the opinions of the developers and their profession-specific biases.

Outcome-based clinical practice guidelines include a measure of the effectiveness of evidence-based recommendations within the guidelines, evaluating whether the recommendation improved the quality of care. Various methods, such as meta-analysis, decision analysis, or cost-effectiveness analysis, may be used to determine the effectiveness of the recommendation.

The rarest type of clinical practice guidelines is preference-based. Here, evidence-based and outcome-based guidelines are combined with patient preferences for possible outcomes of the interventions. The inclusion of patient preferences makes these guidelines very difficult to create, but these are the only guidelines that take into account the variability in individual patients' values and include the patients' values in the decision-making process.

In the past five years, a growing interest in evidence-based clinical practice guidelines has developed among North American health practitioners. Consequently, several evidence-based clinical practice guidelines that are relevant to the management of certain types of musculoskeletal conditions have been published, including:

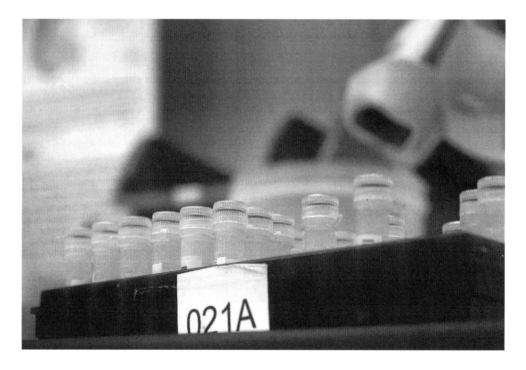

- the guidelines of the Quebec Task Force on Spinal Disorders (1987);
- the Agency for Health Care Policy and Research guidelines for acute low-back pain (1994);
- the British medical journal Clinical Evidence (1999);
- the Philadelphia Panel (2001) for low-back, neck, knee, and shoulder pain;
- the American College of Rheumatology (1995) guidelines for knee osteoarthritis; and
- the Colorado Treatment Guidelines (2006).

In addition, Canadian health practitioners developed their own evidence-based clinical practice guidelines on spinal manipulations and suctioning (College of Physiotherapists of Ontario 1998). The target users of these guidelines are physical therapists, occupational therapists, chiropractors, physiatrists, orthopedic surgeons, rheumatologists, family physicians, and neurologists.

CHAPTER 2: COMMONLY USED THERAPEUTIC MODALITIES

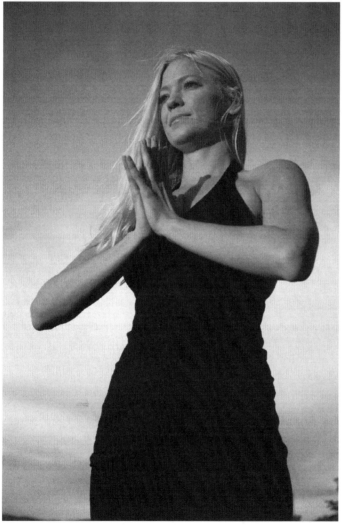

The American Medical Association Current Procedural Terminology manual (2007) defines a modality as any physical agent applied to produce therapeutic changes to biologic tissues, including thermal, acoustic, light, mechanical, or electric energy. Therapeutic modalities are adjunctive treatments to exercise and manual therapy; the use of modalities alone is not considered a form of therapeutic intervention. Modalities may be supervised, not requiring direct patient contact by the provider, or modalities may require constant attendance by a health-care professional. The ultimate goal of a therapeutic intervention is to improve the long-term function of the patient. Decisions regarding the treatment of an individual patient depend on the expertise of the therapist, the equipment available, and the desires of the attending physician. Consequently, a working knowledge of the uses and limitations of different modalities will assist physicians in appropriately prescribing physical agents.

Current Evidence Based Protocols on the use of Therapeutic Modalities

Commonly Used Therapeutic Modalities (Rand et al. 2007)

Modality	Description	Potential Therapeutic Uses
Ultrasound	High-frequency waves are used to warm superficial soft tissues or to accelerate tissue healing at the cellular level.	Tendon injuries, fracture healing, short-term pain relief of muscle strain or spasm
Sonophoresis/ Phonophoresis	Ultrasound is used to deliver therapeutic medications to tissue under the skin.	Inflammatory conditions such as tendonitis, arthritis, and bursitis
Iontophoresis	Electric current is used to deliver ionically charged substances through the skin to deeper tissues.	Calcific tendinopathy, inflammatory conditions, hyperhidrosis
Low-level laser therapy	Photon radiation is applied, altering cellular oxidative metabolism and decreasing prostaglandin E2 concentration.	Minor musculoskeletal pain, carpal tunnel syndrome, osteoarthritis, rheumatoid arthritis
Vertebral axial decompression/ traction	Force expands the intervertebral space and reduces disc protrusion and intradiscal pressure.	Chronic low-back pain
Electrical stimulation	Electric current generates an action potential in nerve tissue, causing a muscle contraction or altering sensory input.	Muscle spasm or contusion (electronic muscle stimulation), neuropathic pain (TENS)

Therapeutic Exercise

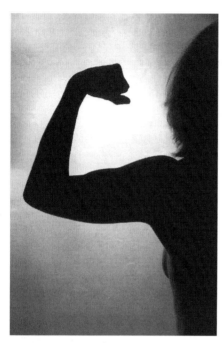

Exercises that target muscle deficiencies or that help rehabilitate patients after surgery or injury are major parts of many protocols. Therapeutic exercise, such as concentric, eccentric, isometric, and isotonic exercises, is used to improve strength, mobility, and function and to decrease pain and swelling. Physicians often prescribe home-based rehabilitation exercises by providing patients with brief instruction and handouts.

Studies have found that home-based therapeutic exercise is beneficial for postoperative recovery after anterior cruciate ligament reconstruction. In contrast, supervised therapeutic exercise has been found to be more beneficial than home-based exercise in patients with low-back injury and osteoarthritis of the knee (Rand et al. 2007).

Ultrasound

Ultrasound (including phonophoresis) uses sonic generators to deliver acoustic energy for therapeutic thermal and/or nonthermal soft-tissue effects. Indications include scar tissue, adhesions, collagen fiber and muscle spasm, and the need to extend muscle tissue or accelerate the soft-tissue healing. Ultrasound with electrical stimulation is the concurrent delivery of electrical energy that involves dispersive electrode placement. Indications include muscle spasm, scar tissue, pain modulation, and muscle facilitation. Phonophoresis is the transfer of medication to the target tissue to control inflammation and pain through the use of sonic generators. These topical medications include, but are not limited to, steroidal anti-inflammatory, and anesthetics. Positive effects should be noted at around six to fifteen treatments. Patients should be seen three times per week. The optimum duration is four to eight weeks. The maximum duration of the program is two months (State of Colorado 2006).

Ultrasound has many medical applications, including those that are diagnostic, operative, and therapeutic. It has been used therapeutically for more than half a century and is currently one of the most widely and frequently used electrotherapeutic modalities.

Ultrasound is a form of acoustic (sound) energy with a frequency above the limit detectable by the human ear. The acoustic energy generated from ultrasound is produced by a piezoelectric crystal within a transducer, which emits high-frequency acoustic pressure waves (1 to 12 MHz) that are transmitted through body tissues by molecular vibrations and collisions. Therapeutic ultrasound consists of high-frequency vibrations that can be pulsed or continuous. High-intensity focused ultrasound, which directs high-intensity acoustic energy within a tissue to increase the heat produced by the waves as they are absorbed by the tissue, increases the temperature in local tissues (Claps and Willie 2007). At lower intensities, however, where there is virtually no increase in local temperature, ultrasound has been shown to be beneficial to fracture healing. This lower-intensity ultrasound is referred to as low-intensity pulsed ultrasound (Claes and Willie 2007, Speed 2001, Molizoset 2006).

Therapeutic ultrasound is commonly used in the treatment of musculoskeletal injury to increase tissue temperature and increase healing rates. Based on their meta-analysis of trials of treatments for soft-tissue lesions of the shoulder, the research concluded that ultrasound is not effective and its use should be discouraged. This conclusion was later criticized as being based on methodologically inadequate research studies. The criticisms emphasized the need for double-blind studies, an internally valid method of placebo treatment. An adequate group size and details of the dosage of ultrasound used are also needed (Robertson and Baker 2001).

It is also important to identify the clinical problems for which ultrasound is anecdotally effective. Low-intensity ultrasound has shown tremendous promise as a treatment for delayed unions and nonunions and as a method to facilitate distraction osteogenesis and bone graft incorporation (Khan and Laurencin 2008). The three most common impairments ultrasound manages are soft-tissue inflammation (e.g., bursitis, tendinitis; 83.6%), tissue extensibility (71%), and scar-tissue remodeling (69%) (Wong et al. 2007). Consequently, the use of ultrasound in therapeutics has gained prominence in recent years, evidenced by the increase in patents filed and new commercial devices launched.

Benefits in Fracture Healing

While advances in the operative and nonoperative care of fractures continue to improve patient outcomes, even under the best of circumstances recovery times often take months. This can have profound personal and economic consequences for patients and their families. Five to 10% of the 5.6 million fractures that occur annually in the United States are complicated by delayed healing or nonunion (Busse et al. 2002). For example, the tibia is the most commonly fractured long bone and accounts for 35–65% of all nonunions. This has substantial economic impact when one considers repeat surgery and prolonged therapy in treating these fractures. The need to decrease health-care spending has led to interest in modalities that can enhance and hasten healing of fractures, diminish the incidence of nonunions, and, in the event of delayed or nonunion, treat them effectively.

Many modalities have been used in an attempt to accelerate fracture healing and prevent delayed or nonunions, including ultrasound. Extracorporeal shock-wave therapy (orthotripsy) has been used in the treatment of nonunions, under the premise that these high-energy waves cause microfractures of the bone trabeculae and this tissue damage encourages the reparative process leading to fracture union. Prospective studies with more than 700 patients have reported healing success rates of 62–83%. However, the practicality of this treatment is questionable because it is painful and requires anesthesia and often hospital admission.

As a result of continuing research into better methods of external stimulation of fracture healing, low-intensity (temporally averaged intensity of less than 0.1 W/cm2) pulsed ultrasound has emerged as a safe and effective modality to enhance fracture healing. With low-intensity ultrasound, heat generation at the soft tissue-bone interface has been shown to be insignificant. Similarly, the risk for tissue-damaging inertial cavitation is negligible. As with shock-wave treatment, low-intensity ultrasound is applied externally; however, it is painless and can be applied on a daily basis in the patient's home. In contrast, high-intensity (1.0 to 2 W/cm2) continuous ultrasound was deleterious to fracture healing in animal studies, and it posed a considerable risk for tissue damage.

In October 1994 the US Food and Drug Administration (FDA) approved the use of ultrasound in fresh fractures and subsequently approved its use for established nonunions in February 2000 (Rubin et al. 2001). A number of prospective, randomized, double-blind, placebo-controlled trials have demonstrated the efficacy of ultrasound in accelerating fracture healing.

Heckman et al. (1994) evaluated tibial fractures in a prospective randomized study in which low-intensity pulsed ultrasound (consisting of a burst width of 200 msec containing 1.5 MHz sine waves, with a repetition rate of 1 kHz) was applied for twenty minutes per day until there was radiographic evidence of three healed cortices. Thirty-three patients with a mean age of thirty-six were in the experimental group, while thirty-four patients with a mean age of thirty-one were in the placebo group.

Favorable results were shown with ultrasound treatment. There was a statistically significant decrease in time to clinical healing, with a mean of eighty-six days in the ultrasound group compared with 114 days in the control group. There were no serious complications from ultrasound use, and patient compliance with the ultrasound device was excellent.

Gebauer et al. (2005) examined the effects of low-intensity pulsed ultrasound on nonunions and found that 85% of nonunions healed after a twenty-minute daily transdermal treatment, which matched the healing rates achieved after surgical intervention. Kristiansen et al. (1997) reported a multicenter clinical trial in which they showed the efficacy of ultrasound in accelerating healing of distal radial fractures. There was a significant difference in time to union with the use of ultrasound, with the ultrasound group healing in sixty-one days compared with the placebo group healing in ninety-eight days. Specifically, at forty-two days after the fracture, 20% of thirty fractures treated with the active device healed compared with 3% of fractures treated with the placebo device.

Results similar to those of Heckman et al. (1994) and Kristiansen et al. (1997) were shown by Mayr et al. (2000) in healing fresh scaphoid fractures. Fractures treated with ultrasound healed in forty-three days compared with sixty-two days in the control group.

These studies demonstrate that, among the modalities available to enhance fracture healing, ultrasound is a safe, practical, and effective treatment. Specialized ultrasound units (e.g., the Exogen 2000+) have been developed to treat fractured bone. Although these units are highly efficacious, their cost is high because the units are leased on a patient-to-patient basis rather than purchased by individual clinics (Warden et al. 2006). A significant beneficial effect of low-intensity pulsed ultrasound produced by conventional therapeutic ultrasound units on fracture repair has been demonstrated. However, before the use of conventional units can be contemplated, therapists need to be aware of the variability in the output performance of ultrasound units.

Equipment surveys undertaken globally have found that many ultrasound units used in clinical practice are unable to produce an ultrasound dose that matches the metered dose to a point within set standards (Hekkenberg et al. 2001). This output variance may not only influence treatment efficacy during fracture repair, but it may also elicit detrimental effects. Unless these current limitations are addressed, the use of conventional therapeutic ultrasound units in a manner other than that approved by the US FDA could have potential negative ramifications.

Mechanism of Action

Despite the overwhelmingly positive clinical data supporting low-intensity pulsed ultrasound as a treatment for fracture repair, the exact mechanism through which the treatment proves beneficial is still largely unknown. Ultrasound is likely to influence each key stage of fracture healing: inflammation, repair, and remodeling. Moreover, ultrasound has been shown to affect angiogenesis, chondrogenesis, and osteogenesis.

Potential Mechanisms of Low-Intensity Pulsed Ultrasound Effect on Fracture Healing
• Mechanical signal transduction and induction of gene expression • Activation of enzymes in response to heat energy • Increased vascularity at the fracture site • Modulation of intracellular calcium signaling • Enhanced cartilage calcification and maturation

To gain a better understanding of how low-intensity pulsed ultrasound affects bone as it is repaired, Leung et al. (2004) used low-intensity pulsed ultrasound in patients with open tibial fractures and high-energy complex fractures and found a 42% acceleration in healing over non-low-intensity pulsed-ultrasound-treated fractures. Interestingly, Leung et al. (2004) went on to evaluate patient plasma levels of bone-specific alkaline phosphatase, a well-characterized phenotypic marker of osteoblast differentiation, and found increases in its levels in patients receiving low-intensity pulsed ultrasound. This finding supported the idea that the mode of effectiveness of low-intensity pulsed ultrasound was at the cellular level.

Mechanism of Fracture Healing

In order to understand the mechanism of ultrasound action on fracture healing, it is important to first understand the mechanism of fracture healing. Fracture healing is a form of wound repair and is driven by the recruitment of cells and the expression of genes. As mentioned above, it is generally divided into three stages: inflammatory, reparative, and remodeling. The inflammatory stage commences with the disruption of blood vessels from the injury and the formation of a hematoma. Inflammatory cells invade the hematoma and initiate lysosomal degradation of necrotic tissue (Hadjiargyrou 1998).

The reparative phase begins within four to five days following the fracture. Pluripotential mesenchymal stem cells invade the area and differentiate into fibroblasts, chondroblasts, and osteoblasts. These cells are responsible for the formation of a soft fracture callus and the subsequent formation of woven bone. Angiogenesis within the marrow cavity and the periosteal tissue helps to deliver the appropriate cells to the fracture site. Cartilage cells are present in the fracture site as early as five days postinjury, and the soft callus is formed, stabilizing the fractured ends of the bone. The process of osteoid formation, mineralization, and creation of woven bone then begins (Hadjiargyrou 1998).

The final stage in the process of fracture healing is the remodeling stage, which can continue up to several years following the fracture. Fracture callus is remodeled from immature woven bone into mature lamellar bone. The end result is mature lamellar bone oriented along lines of stress, thereby creating normal or near-normal morphology and strength without a scar.

The definition of a delayed union is generally thought to be healing not completed by three months. Of these delayed unions, some will still remain "un-united" at nine months postfracture and are thus classified as nonunions (Hadjiargyrou 1998).

Cellular Reaction

The biophysical effects of ultrasound are traditionally separated into thermal and nonthermal effects, although according to Baker et al. (2001) it is incorrect to assume that only one effect is present at any time and that treatment may be classed as either thermal (i.e., continuous wave exposure) or nonthermal (i.e., pulsed exposure).

Pulsing the ultrasound beam reduces the rise in temperature proportionately to the pulsing ratio; it does not eliminate the heating. In addition, although low-intensity pulsed ultrasound results in a less than 1°C increase in local tissue temperature, some local effects have been attributed to this minor change, including increased blood flow and the stimulation of enzymatic activity such as that of matrix metalloproteinase-1, which is known to be sensitive to very small temperature changes.

As ultrasound waves pass through tissues, absorption of the waves is proportionate to the density of the tissue. This may explain how ultrasound therapy can be targeted to the fracture gap, since bone is of greater density than the surrounding soft tissues. Therefore, the cells themselves may sense this mechanical alteration in their environment and must then translate this change into a molecular response, thus modulating cell function. As a result, it is best to assume that nonthermal effects will always be accompanied by some heating and that acoustic fields that give rise to heating are always accompanied by nonthermal effects (Baker et al. 2001).

Studies at the cellular level when low-intensity pulsed ultrasound is applied to a fracture site have shown evidence of increased extracellular collagen synthesis, modifications in integrin expression, and intracellular events such as increased cell proliferation, cell differentiation, protein and factor synthesis, gene expression, and alterations in cytosolic Ca2+ levels, to name just a few. There is evidence to suggest that ultrasound stimulates osteogenesis through calcium signaling and calcification of cartilage.

There is no direct evidence that any purported clinical benefits of ultrasound are due to altered membrane permeability. The only experimental evidence for ultrasonically altered membrane permeability comes from studies of cell cultures for which there was good evidence that cavitation occurred. Cavitation is the formation of tiny gas bubbles in the tissues because of ultrasound vibration. Gas bubbles have the potential to oscillate and cause damage under the influence of ultrasound.

Benefits in Osteoarthritis

A recent Cochrane report (Rutjes et al. 2010) compared therapeutic ultrasound with sham or no specific intervention in terms of effects on pain and function and safety outcomes in patients with knee or hip osteoarthritis and concluded that therapeutic ultrasound may be beneficial for patients with osteoarthritis of the knee. Osteoarthritis is an age-related disease of the joints characterized by focal areas of loss of articular cartilage in synovial joints, accompanied by subchondral bone changes, osteophyte formation at the joint margins, thickening of the joint capsule, and mild synovitis. The objectives of management of knee and hip osteoarthritis are to relieve pain and to maintain or improve function. People who used therapeutic ultrasound had an improvement in their pain of about three on a scale from zero (no pain) to ten (extreme pain) after using it for two months. No adverse events or withdrawals due to adverse events occurred in the trials.

Benefits in Soft-Tissue Shoulder Disorders

Shoulder pain is a major reason that patients seek consultations with physicians. Pain resulting from soft-tissue damage restricts range of motion (ROM) and limits daily activities. According to the recommendation of the Philadelphia Panel (an expert panel on selected rehabilitation interventions for shoulder pain), ultrasound therapy is an acceptable physical therapy intervention for shoulder pain. Increased blood flow, increased vascular permeability, increased cell metabolism, enhancement of fibrous tissue extensibility, and muscle relaxation are the purported physiologic effects of ultrasound therapy. A recent systematic review of the published literature has revealed beneficial effects of ultrasound for the treatment of soft-tissue shoulder injury or pain (Alexander et al. 2010). However, the beneficial effects of ultrasound were dependent on length of exposure times and the number of treatment sessions.

The study aimed to systematically and critically review available literature to ascertain whether beneficial effects of ultrasound were associated with certain shoulder pathologies or particular ultrasound treatment protocols. Eight randomized controlled trials that utilized ultrasound for soft-tissue shoulder injury or pain were included in the analysis. The intensity of ultrasound used varied greatly among the studies. In addition, the mean application time per treatment session and the number of treatment sessions also varied, ranging from 4.5 to 15.8 minutes per treatment session and from six to thirty-nine treatment sessions. Studies that showed beneficial effects typically had four times longer total exposure times and applied much greater ultrasound energy per session. Furthermore, when insufficient ultrasound energy (e.g., less than 720 J per session) was provided, positive outcomes were rarely observed.

Variations in the treatment intensity, duration, frequency, and location of ultrasound applications could explain the limited effectiveness of ultrasound therapy in soft-tissue disorders of the shoulder reported in previous studies, which found little evidence that active therapeutic ultrasound is more effective than placebo for treating individuals with shoulder pain (Gursel et al. 2004). Recently, both low-level laser therapy and manual acupuncture were reported to be more effective than ultrasound in treating patients with subacromial impingement syndrome (Santamato et al. 2009, Johansson et al. 2005). Like ultrasound, low-level laser therapy and acupuncture are common interventions, often used in combination with other modalities such as exercise. These findings suggest that future primary studies must focus on selecting optimal ultrasound parameters that deliver more than 720 joules of ultrasound energy per session and treatment schedules that expose tissues to ultrasound for a sufficient period of time (average exposure time of greater than five hours) and evaluate the treatment regimen in randomized, placebo-controlled trials.

High-Intensity Ultrasound

Not all effects of ultrasound on tissue are beneficial. Ultrasound delivered at 1 W/cm2 and a 1 MHz frequency, similar to a treatment that is given to break up kidney stones, has been shown to increase the temperature in the human gastrocnemius muscle by 0.2°C per minute. Although the rise in temperature can be beneficial, such as for pain relief for ligament injuries like tennis elbow, the addition of excessive energy to tissue poses potential risks. For example, bone damage, including inhibition of bone growth and damage to bone marrow has been shown to occur in dogs at intensities above 3 W/cm2. Thus, ultrasound used inappropriately may be at best ineffective or at worst damaging to the patient.

Factors Affecting the Transmission of Acoustic Energy

Due to its potential beneficial and deleterious effects, both of which depend on the intensity and duration of application, the ultrasound sound-head output should be what is expected. Researchers have reported that a large number of therapeutic ultrasound machines used clinically were not within the standard. More than one-third of machines tested in a study by Artho et al. (2002) were outside the standard for power output, and approximately one-fourth of the mechanical times were outside the standard. FDA guidelines regulate the accuracy of the output power produced, permitting a plus or minus 20% error band, and the FDA requires that manufacturers report an error band for effective radiating area (ERA) but stop short of dictating what an acceptable percentage of error is. Most manufacturers report a plus or minus 20% error for ERA; few manufacturers report actual measured ERA value for each transducer. A manufacturer utilizing a combination of plus or minus 20% ERA and plus or minus 20% W permits a theoretical minimum-to-maximum spatial average intensity range of 150% between ultrasound heads while remaining in compliance with FDA guidelines. Even small differences in spatial average intensity have the potential to cause changes in tissue heating (Straub et al. 2008).

Based on the heating rates published by Draper et al. (1995), if a clinician planned to provide a 1 MHz ultrasound treatment at 1.0W/cm2 for ten minutes with the goal of increasing tissue temperature by 1.5°C, the use of Mettler transducer #486 might evoke a temperature rise close to 2.5°C. In contrast, the use of Mettler transducer #167 would likely evoke a rise greater than 3.4°C. These differences would greatly influence tissue response, as the heating levels progressed from a desired level of mild heating to vigorous heating. Thus, further improvements in the accuracy of ultrasound machine calibration are needed. Manufacturers must take more care in reporting proper ERA values. Accurate measures of ERA, output power, spatial average intensity, and energy dosing are critical when developing studies to determine clinical efficacy and attain consistent clinical outcomes while using therapeutic ultrasound.

Tissue healing rates also depend on the conductivity of products used to deliver acoustic energy during ultrasound treatment. Conductivity varies greatly among dressing products. Ultrasound has been used for decades in the management of cutaneous wounds, where it has been shown to accelerate the healing process in incisional lesions, diabetic ulcers, and venous ulcers. The use of adjunctive noncontact ultrasound, operating at a frequency of 40 kHz, appears to improve healing in wounds that fail to heal with conventional wound care alone (Bell and Cavorsi 2008). In addition, noncontact ultrasound significantly decreased wound pain (Bell and Cavorsi 2008). Through-dressing insonation (1-3 MHz) protects the wound from trauma, infection, and heat loss, but it allows the wound bed to be exposed to ultrasound energy. However, if wounds are to be treated through dressings, it is necessary for clinicians to be aware of the ultrasound transmission characteristics of the dressings since different brands of the same type of dressing may have quite different conductivity.

Klucinec et al. (2000) examined the ultrasound conduction and effectiveness of four hydrogel sheets (Nu-Gel, ClearSite, Aquasorb Border, and CarraDres) and four film dressings (CarraSmart Film, J & J Bioclusive, Tegaderm, and Opsite

Flexigrid) used for wound care. Five intensities at a frequency of 3.3 MHz were studied. Nu-Gel was the most efficient hydrogel, and CarraSmart Film was the most efficient film dressing. Thus, conduction of products used to deliver acoustic energy during ultrasound of wounds varies greatly among dressing products and should be considered when selecting a dressing.

Phonophoresis

Ultrasound may be used to increase the penetration of pharmacologically active drugs, usually analgesics or steroids, through the skin to deeper tissues. This technique is known as sonophoresis or phonophoresis. It is used for the treatment of conditions that may also be treated with local anesthetics or steroid injections. Sonophoresis has been shown to increase skin permeability to various low- and high-molecule-weight drugs, including insulin and heparin. There is a risk of thermal injury, however, which increases with the amount and intensity of the energy applied (Hecox et al. 1994).

Based on the systematic review by Hoppenrath and Ciccone (2006), phonophoresis is not more effective than ultrasound in treating pain associated with lateral epicondylitis. Phonophoresis is often used to enhance the transdermal administration of certain medications such as an anti-inflammatory steroid or nonsteroidal anti-inflammatory drug (NSAID). A corticosteroid or nonsteroidal anti-inflammatory drug is usually mixed with an appropriate aqueous base in a 10% concentration and is applied with ultrasound at 1–2W/cm2. This systematic review analyzed trials that used hydrocortisone phonophoresis and compared it with traditional ultrasound therapy.

Phonophoretic research often suffers from poor calibration in terms of the amount of ultrasound energy emitted, and therefore current research must focus on the safety of exposure to ultrasound and miniaturization of devices in order to make this technology a commercial reality. More research is needed to identify the role of various parameters influencing sonophoresis/phonophoresis so that the process can be optimized.

Iontophoresis

Iontophoresis is the transfer of medication, including steroidal anti-inflammatories and anesthetics, into tissue through the use of electrical stimulation. Indications include pain (lidocaine), inflammation (hydrocortisone, salicylate), edema (mecholyl, hyaluronidase, and salicylate), ischemia (magnesium, mecholyl, and iodine), muscle spasm (magnesium, calcium), calcific deposits (acetate), and scars and keloids (chlorine, iodine, acetate). Positive effects should be noted at around one to four treatments. Patients should be seen three times per week with at least forty-eight hours between treatments. The optimum duration is four to six weeks. The maximum duration of the program is six weeks (State of Colorado 2006).

This modality uses an electric current to deliver an ionically charged substance through the skin to deeper tissues. Described initially by Le Duc in 1908, iontophoresis is often used to treat arthritis, bursitis, and tendinopathy. It can also be used to treat hyperhidrosis and certain dermatophytoses. Dexamethasone 0.4% solution is the most commonly prescribed medication used to treat tendinopathies and possible inflammatory conditions. Cathodes are used for negatively charged substances, and anodes are used for positively charged substances. The amperage used depends on the natural resistance provided by the skin.

Iontophoresis, in conjunction with traditional modalities, can shorten treatment time for plantar fasciitis. One small study found that acetic acid iontophoresis in conjunction with ultrasound was beneficial in the treatment of myositis ossificans (Wieder 1992). Myositis ossificans is characterized by heterotopic ossification (calcification) of muscle. Calcification usually appears within two to three weeks. The acetate ion found in acetic acid is negative in polarity and has been cited as effective in reducing the size of calcium deposits through the absorption of calcium. Because recurrent injury resulting in additional bleeding is often a precursor to the myositis ossificans formation, additional damage to tissues and resultant bleeding may occur from invasive injection by a syringe and needle.

Low-Level Laser Therapy

Laser therapy is based on the idea that laser radiation is able to alter cellular and tissue functions in a manner that is dependent on the characteristics of the light itself (i.e., its wavelength). By definition, low-level laser therapy (often also known as "low-energy" or "low-power" laser therapy) refers to the use of red-beam or near-infrared lasers with a wavelength between 600–1000 nm and power from 5–500 mW. In contrast, lasers employed in surgery typically use 300 W. Low-level laser therapy emits no heat, sound, or vibration. Therefore, it is assumed that any biologic effects are secondary to the direct effect of photonic radiation or photochemical reactions in the cells, also referred to as photobiology or biostimulation.

Low-level laser therapy is approved by the US FDA for the treatment of hand and wrist pain associated with carpal tunnel syndrome and for minor musculoskeletal pain. In addition, low-level laser therapy has been advocated for use in a wide range of medical conditions including wound healing, temporomandibular joint disorders (TMJ), lateral and medial epicondylitis, osteoarthritis, and rheumatoid arthritis. Although nausea has been reported with prolonged use, there are no other known adverse effects. Low-level laser therapy can be administered by physicians, chiropractors, physical therapists, and occupational therapists. It is generally provided in an office where no anesthesia or sedation is needed.

Laser radiation may alter cell and tissue function. Laboratory studies suggest that radiation stimulates collagen production, alters DNA synthesis, and improves the function of damaged neurological tissue. A single dose of low-level laser therapy improved the normalized ultimate tensile strength (UTS) and stiffness of the laser-treated group significantly more than control with placebo laser (Fung et al. 2002).

Although the mechanism for low-level laser therapy is not well understood, it appears to be related to a photochemical reaction at the cellular level rather than a thermal effect at the cellular level. Cytochrome oxidase acts as an acceptor of photon radiation in the 600–900 nm range. This stimulation increases adenosine triphosphate (ATP) production and cellular oxidative metabolism.

One proposed animal model is that low-level laser therapy enhances the action of superoxide dismutase, which prevents the proliferation of prostaglandin E. A recent study showed a significant decrease in prostaglandin E2 concentration in peritendinous fluid treated with low-level laser therapy versus sham therapy. This suggests that the effects of low-level laser therapy may be mediated by decreased prostaglandin synthesis. Larger studies are needed, however, to confirm this mechanism.

Trials on the efficacy of low-level laser therapy have been systematically reviewed for rheumatoid arthritis (Brousseau et al. 2005). Six studies with a total of 220 patients with rheumatoid arthritis were included in the review. The experimental and placebo groups in the reviewed studies showed a significant difference, suggesting that low-level laser therapy is effective for increasing range of motion and reducing rheumatoid arthritis-related pain and morning stiffness. Further studies are needed to determine the optimal wavelength, dosage, application techniques, and duration of intervention and to determine long-term effects in patients with rheumatoid arthritis.

A similar Cochrane review of low-level laser therapy in patients with osteoarthritis showed minimal improvement in pain and joint movement (Brousseau et al. 2005). The review included seven controlled clinical trials with 184 patients randomized to laser and 161 patients randomized to an inactive laser probe. However, other reviews that were not conducted systematically did not yield reports of any effect of low-intensity laser therapy for musculoskeletal pain relief. In general, low-level laser therapy has not been shown to cause adverse effects, but a benefit has not been clearly established.

Some systematic reviews and randomized clinical trials have suggested that low-level laser therapy could be an effective intervention for decreasing chronic low-back pain. Although low-level laser therapy may improve pain and functional disability in chronic low-back pain, it does not bring any additional benefits to exercise therapy.

Laser therapy treatment times are usually ten to twenty minutes per session. Chronic low-back pain patients will usually respond best to three to four treatments per week. Maximum effect is often reached in three to four weeks, but several months of care may be necessary in extremely complex cases. It is important to allow time for delayed effects and cumulative effects, which may be necessary in extremely complex cases. While laser therapies can often produce results as a stand-alone therapy, they also work very well adjunctively with other therapies such as physical therapy, manipulation, exercise, and stretching. The wound-healing effects of therapeutic lasers are a valuable adjunct during postoperative recovery.

Differences in studies of low-level laser therapy (i.e., device used, end points, control group) make it difficult to determine the effectiveness of this modality. In general, low-level laser therapy has not been shown to cause adverse effects, but a benefit has not been clearly established.

Electrical Stimulation

There are several electrical stimulation methods used in therapy. These include electrical muscle stimulation and transcutaneous (through the skin) electrical nerve stimulation (TENS).

Functional electrical stimulation is an accepted treatment in which electrical current is applied to elicit involuntary or assisted contractions of atrophied and/or impaired muscles. It may be indicated for muscle atrophy due to radiculopathy.
The time to produce effect is two to six treatments three times per week with a maximum duration of eight weeks. If beneficial, the patient can be provided with a home unit (State of Colorado 2006).

Manual electrical stimulation is used for peripheral nerve injuries or pain reduction that requires continuous application or supervision or involves extensive teaching. Indications include muscle spasm (including TENS), atrophy, decreased circulation, osteogenic stimulation, inflammation, and the need to facilitate muscle hypertrophy, muscle strengthening, muscle responsiveness in spinal cord injury/brain injury (SCI/BI), and peripheral neuropathies. It is recommended to be used three to seven times per week with a maximum duration of two months (State of Colorado 2006).

Unattended electrical stimulation, once applied, requires minimal on-site supervision by the physical or nonphysical provider. Indications include pain, inflammation, muscle spasm, atrophy, decreased circulation, and the need for osteogenic stimulation. A TENS home unit should be purchased if treatment is effective and frequent use is recommended. Positive effects should be noted at around two to four treatments (State of Colorado 2006).

Electrical Stimulation, Percutaneous (PENS) uses needles to deliver low-voltage electrical current under the skin. Theoretically, this therapy prevents pain signals traveling through small nerve fibers from reaching the brain, similar to the theory of TENS. There is good evidence (Jenner 1995) that PENS produces improvement of pain and function compared to placebo; however, there is no evidence (Jordan and O'Dowd 2011) that the effect is prolonged after the initial three-week treatment episode. There are no well-executed studies (Koes et al. 2001) that show PENS performs better than TENS for chronic-pain patients. PENS is more invasive, requires a trained health-care provider, and has no clear long-term effect; therefore, it is not generally recommended. Positive effects should be noted at around one to four treatments. Patients should be seen two to three times per week. The maximum duration of the program is twelve sessions per year (State of Colorado 2006).

TENS should include least one instructional session for proper application and use. Indications include muscle spasm, atrophy, and decreased circulation and pain control. Minimal TENS unit parameters should include pulse rate, pulse width, and amplitude modulation. The optimum duration is three sessions.

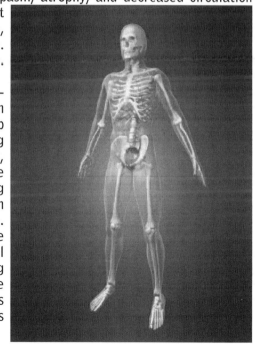

Electrical stimulation uses high-voltage pulsed galvanic stimulation to cause a single muscle or a group of muscles to contract. By placing electrodes on the skin in various locations, the health practitioner can recruit the appropriate muscle fibers. Contracting the muscle via electrical stimulation helps strengthen the affected muscle. The health practitioner can change the current setting to allow for a forceful or gentle muscle contraction. Along with increasing muscle strength, the contraction of the muscle also promotes blood supply to the area, which assists in healing (Gregory and Bickel 2005).

Use of electrical stimulation should be limited to the initial stages of treatment, such as the first week after injury, so that patients may quickly progress to more active treatment that includes a restoration of ROM and strengthening. Electrical stimulation may often be combined with ice or heat to enhance its analgesic effects. The use of electrical stimulation and shoulder taping, in conjunction with other rehabilitation, may play a role in reducing shoulder subluxation (Peterson 2004).

A transcutaneous electrical nerve stimulation unit is a small battery-operated machine that uses electrical transmission to decrease pain. The health practitioner applies electrode patches to the skin over the affected area. The machine is turned on, and a mild electric current is sent from the stationary stimulator through these electrode patches. This signal disrupts the pain signal that is being sent from the affected area to the surrounding nerves. By breaking the signal, the machine allows the patient to experience less pain. The treatment is also believed to stimulate the body's production of endorphins, natural painkillers.

Success rates vary greatly due to many factors, including electrode placement, chronicity of the problem, and previous treatments. Documentation of greater than 50% reduction in pain with a treatment trial may help substantiate electrical stimulation's true beneficial effects as opposed to a placebo response. All in all, more evidence is needed on the long-term benefits, ideal parameters, and overall effectiveness of electrical stimulation methods.

Although the transcutaneous electrical nerve stimulation units can be purchased or rented, a prescription from a physician is required. The health practitioner is often the person to teach the patient how to use the device, including the proper placement of electrodes for optimal benefits.

Although there are few risks with electrical therapy, potential adverse effects primarily include burns from improper parameter settings, allergic reaction to electrodes or the conduction medium, and pain during treatment. Patients with pacemakers should avoid transcutaneous electrical nerve stimulation because the electrical current could interfere with the pacemaker's operation.

Spinal Decompression Therapy

Spinal decompression is one modality that has attempted to address the need for nonsurgical interventions specifically addressing low-back pain of discogenic origin. Approximately 25% of adults in the United States report having experienced low-back pain, and the proportion of physician visits attributed to back pain has changed little since the 1990s. Low-back pain is among the top ten reasons for visits to internists and the most common and most expensive reason for work disability in the United States. It is also a frequent cause of medically related early retirement.

Intervertebral discs, facet joints, ligaments, fascia, muscles, and nerve-root dura have all been identified as structures that can cause pain in the low back. Only abnormalities of the facet joints, intervertebral discs, and sacroiliac joints have been conclusively demonstrated to be causes of low-back pain with the use of established diagnostic techniques. Discogenic pain most commonly affects the lower back, buttocks, and hips and is likely a result of internal disc degeneration. Discogenic pain may be due to progressive annular breakdown and tearing, which stimulate pain fibers in the outer one-third of the annulus.

Many alternatives are available for the management of low-back pain, but little consensus has been established on which options are appropriate or preferable for various scenarios. The three major categories of treatment of low-back pain are surgical, nonsurgical, and pharmacologic. Surgical intervention, often with fusion, is frequently suggested for the treatment of discogenic pain, but the end result can be reduced mobility, stiffness, and continuing pain—the "failed-back syndrome." In addition, surgery is associated with risks, and the outcome in many patients with discogenic back pain is unpredictable. In general, if patients do not respond well to exercise and conservative pharmacologic treatment with NSAIDs, nonsurgical, noninvasive therapies (spinal decompression, TENS, acupuncture) are the most frequently and appropriately prescribed.

Various nonsurgical therapies have been developed to achieve decompression in patients with low-back pain, beginning with simple manual traction in which the therapist exerts traction by using the patient's arms and/or legs. Additional types of traction in use today include motorized, mechanical, manual, auto, gravity-dependent (or inverted-suspension), pneumatic, continuous, intermittent, bed-rest, and underwater traction. These types of traction can be difficult to standardize, however, because of potential fatigue on the part of both the patient and therapist or the patient's inability to tolerate the force or the position.

With respect to neck or back applications, traction can be defined as an intermittent or continuous force applied along the long axis of the spine in an attempt to elongate the spine, or the act of pulling or stretching muscle or joints. This, in turn, may facilitate oxygen and nutrient uptake and improve disc metabolism and restoration. Experimental data exist to support the concept that traction can expand the intervertebral space and reduce disc protrusion and intradiscal pressure. However, the results of systematic reviews are conflicting, and pain relief with traction has been inconsistent and short-lived.

A randomized study that compared traction in a semi-reclined position at a 30-degree angle with exercise versus exercise alone found little difference between the two modalities, leading the authors to conclude that traction has no effect beyond that of the normal regimen (Boman et al. 2003). Moreover, a recent meta-analysis found that very few randomized, placebo-controlled trials evaluating traction reported positive effects on low-back pain; instead, increased pain and intervertebral pressure have been reported after its use (Clark et al. 2007).

Devices Currently on the Market

Motorized traction devices that purport to produce nonsurgical disc decompression by creating negative intradiscal pressure in the disc space include devices with the trade names of DRX 9000 and VAX-D.

DRX9000

Spinal decompression with the DRX9000 computerized, nonsurgical spinal decompression system was designed to provide maximum patient benefits with the use of a noninvasive approach that may help minimize health-care resources and offer a potentially optimal therapeutic approach to the treatment of low-back pain. Spinal decompression has the capability of relieving pressure on the spinal nerves caused by disc herniation and degenerative disc disease and is helpful for conditions such as sciatica and facet syndrome.

Several studies have demonstrated the efficacy of spinal decompression therapy. In a recent study of 219 patients with herniated discs and degenerative disc disease, 86% who completed the therapy showed immediate improvement and resolution of their symptoms; 92% improved overall; and 2% relapsed within ninety days of initial treatment (Glovis and Groteke 2003).

Vertebral Axial Decompression (VAX-D)

Although the literature demonstrates success for treating herniated discs conservatively, many patients still undergo a surgical procedure to treat their nerve-root compression. Nonsurgical decompression could have significant advantages over the surgical methods currently in use. These include reduced costs, early return to work, lower morbidity, reduced postoperative care, and elimination of the failed-back syndrome.

The vertebral axial decompression (VAX-D) Therapeutic Table is an FDA-approved, computer-controlled motorized traction device used to stretch the back. The device is a two-part table in which the upper part is fixed to the table frame and the lower part slides back and forth to provide intermittent traction. The patient is anchored to the lower part by a pelvic harness.

The VAX-D has demonstrated its effectiveness in treating low-back pain with and without radiculopathy (Beattie et al. 2008). Traction applied in the prone position using the VAX-D for eight weeks was associated with improvements in pain intensity at thirty and 180 days after discharge in a sample of patients with activity-limiting low-back pain and evidence of a degenerative and/or herniated intervertebral disc at one or more levels of the lumbar spine. The table asserts its effect through decompression of the intervertebral disc and has reduced intradiscal pressures to a negative 150 mm Hg. It is assumed that reduction of intradiscal pressures to such significant levels should produce nerve-root decompression, but this has not been specifically investigated.

The single randomized, placebo-controlled trial of spinal decompression therapy (Sherry et al. 2001) compared the VAX-D unit to TENS for the treatment of chronic (greater than three months in duration) low-back pain. The average duration of pain in the study population was 7.3 years, and the average age was forty-two. Treatment consisted of thirty-minute sessions five times per week for four weeks, followed by weekly sessions for four weeks. Outcome measures were the visual analog pain scale (VAS) and an improvement in the level of functioning as measured by patient-nominated disability ratings. Successful outcome was defined as a 50% decrease in pain using the VAS scale.

At the conclusion of the study, the TENS-treated group (n=21) reported a success rate of 0%, while the group treated with VAX-D (n=19) showed a success rate of approximately 69%. It is difficult to conclude from this study that VAX-D is effective for treating chronic back pain, since detailed statistics regarding the outcomes for each group were not included in the analysis. Furthermore, patients were not blinded to the treatment received, thus there may have been a negative placebo effect in the TENS-treated group.

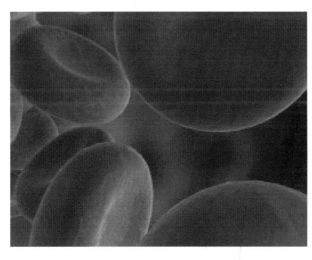

The Australian Medical Services Advisory Committee (2001) performed an assessment of the literature on VAX-D therapy and concluded that there is insufficient evidence regarding the efficacy of the therapy. VAX-D has never been compared to exercise, spinal manipulation, standard medical care, or other less expensive conservative treatment options.

VAX-D therapy is usually provided in an outpatient setting for the purpose of relieving back pain. Its providers—chiropractors, osteopathic physicians, and physical therapists—commonly recommend twenty sessions of thirty to forty-five minutes, with a total cost of several thousand dollars. Ordinary traction, in which a steady stretching force is applied to the pelvis using weights and pulleys, has not been proven effective against back pain. VAX-D's intermittent traction can be effective for pain associated with bulging discs. However, manual manipulation is equally effective. No type of traction has proven effective for herniated discs, which often require surgery.

Proponents of the VAX-D claim that the device can relieve low-back pain by decompressing discs, improving the flow of nutrients into the disc, and rehydrating dried-out discs, thereby helping to restore the disc structure. Even if the VAX-D therapy can lower interdiscal pressure and reduce disk bulging while the patient is on the table, it has not been proven that changes persist after the patient resumes standing.

Proponents also claim that a large study published in 1998 found that VAX-D was 71% effective in reducing pain in patients with degenerated discs, facet syndrome, and sciatica. However, the study was so poorly designed that no conclusions about effectiveness can be drawn from the published report. For example, there was no control group, so it is not possible to determine whether patients improved as a result of treatment or would have recovered without it. The data to enable comparison between VAX-D treatment and other forms of treatment is unavailable. VAX-D treatment is promoted as being completely risk-free.

VAX-D is an expensive high-tech form of mechanical traction that can provide relief in some cases of back pain but is widely promoted with unsubstantiated claims that it can correct degenerated and herniated discs without surgery.

CHAPTER 3: OTHER THERAPEUTIC MODALITIES

Interdisciplinary rehabilitation programs are the gold standard of treatment for individuals with chronic pain who have not responded to less intensive modes of treatment. There is good evidence that interdisciplinary programs will improve function and decrease disability (Bulger et al. 2002).

Interdisciplinary programs evaluate and treat painful musculoskeletal, neurological, and other chronic painful disorders and psychological issues, drug dependence, abuse or addiction, high levels of stress and anxiety, failed surgery, and preexisting or latent psychopathology.

To ensure positive functional outcomes, communication between the patient, insurer, and all professionals involved must be coordinated and consistent. Any exchange of information must involve all parties, including the patient. Care decisions should be communicated to all and should include the family or other support system.

Use of modalities may be early in the process to facilitate compliance with therapeutic exercise, physical conditioning, and increasing functional activities. Active treatments should be emphasized over passive treatments. Active treatments should encourage self-coping skills and management of pain, which can be continued independently at home or at work. Treatments that can foster a sense of dependency by the patient on the caregiver should be avoided. Treatment length should be decided based upon observed functional improvement.

Aerobic conditioning and strengthening are superior to treatment programs that do not include exercise (Clifton et al. 2001). A therapeutic exercise program should be initiated at the start of any treatment rehabilitation. Such programs should emphasize education, independence, and the importance of an ongoing exercise regime. Exercise alone or part of a multidisciplinary program results in decreased disability for workers with non-acute low-back pain. There is no sufficient evidence to support the recommendation of any particular exercise regimen over any other (Clifton 2004).

When return to work is an option, it may be appropriate to implement a Work Hardening Program. For patients currently employed, efforts should be aimed at keeping them employed. Formal rehabilitation programs should provide assistance in creating work profiles.

Patients with pain need to reestablish a healthy balance in lifestyle. All providers should educate patients on how to overcome barriers to resume daily activity, including pain management, decreased energy levels, financial constraints, decreased physical ability, and change in family dynamics.

Acupuncture

Acupuncture is an accepted and widely used procedure for the relief of pain and inflammation (Genovese 2005). The exact mode of action is only partially understood. Western medicine studies suggest that acupuncture stimulates the nervous system at the level of the brain, promotes deep relaxation, and affects the release of neurotransmitters. Acupuncture is commonly used as an alternative or in addition to traditional Western medicine. While it is commonly used when pain medication is reduced or not tolerated, it may be used as an adjunct to physical rehabilitation and/or surgical intervention to hasten the return to functional activity (Genovese 2005).

Acupuncture is the insertion and removal of filiform needles to stimulate acupuncture points. Needles may be inserted, manipulated, and retained for a period of time. Acupuncture can be used to reduce pain, reduce inflammation, increase blood flow, increase range of motion, decrease the side effect of medication-induced nausea, promote relaxation in an anxious patient, and reduce muscle spasm. Indications include joint pain, joint stiffness, soft-tissue pain and inflammation, paresthesia, postsurgical pain relief, muscle spasm, and scar-tissue pain.

Acupuncture with electrical stimulation is the use of electrical current on the needles at the acupuncture site. It is used to increase the effectiveness of the needles by continuous stimulation of the acupuncture point. Physiological effects can include endorphin release for pain relief, reduction of inflammation, increased blood circulation, analgesia through interruption of pain stimulus, and muscle relaxation. Acupuncture with electrical stimulation is indicated to treat chronic pain conditions, pain along a nerve pathway, muscle spasm, inflammation, scar-tissue pain, and pain located in multiple sites.

Acupuncture treatment is based on individual patient needs, and therefore treatment may include a combination of procedures to enhance treatment effect. Other procedures may include the use of heat, soft-tissue manipulation and massage, and exercise.

When acupuncture has been studied in randomized clinical trials (Genovese 2005), it is often compared with sham acupuncture and/or no acupuncture. Because the sham acupuncture interventions in the clinical trials are generally done by trained acupuncturists, and not by totally untrained personnel, the sham acupuncture interventions may include some of the effects of true acupuncture, much as a partial agonist of a drug may produce some of the effects of the actual drug. For example, a sham procedure involving toothpicks rather than acupuncture needles may stimulate cutaneous afferents in spite of not penetrating the skin, much as a neurological sensory examination may test nociceptor function without skin penetration. To the extent that afferent stimulation is part of the mechanism of action of acupuncture, interpreting the sham results as purely a control group would lead to an underestimation of the analgesic effects of acupuncture.

There is good evidence that both acupuncture and sham acupuncture are superior to usual care without acupuncture for moderate short-term and mild long-term alleviation of low-back pain, neck pain, and the pain of joint osteoarthritis. In these studies five to fifteen treatments were provided. Comparisons of acupuncture and sham acupuncture have been inconsistent, and the advantage of

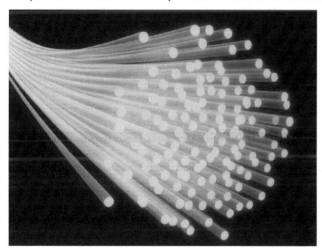

true over sham acupuncture has been small in relation to the advantage of sham over no acupuncture (Genovese 2005).

Acupuncture is an accepted and widely used procedure for the relief of pain and inflammation in cumulative trauma conditions (Genovese 2005). There is some evidence to support its use for lateral epicondylitis (Genovese 2005).

Activities of Daily Living (ADL) Training

Activities of Daily Living (ADL) are well-established interventions that involve instruction, active-assisted training, and/or adaptation of activities or equipment to improve a person's capacity in normal daily activities such as self-care, work reintegration training, homemaking, and driving. ADL (also called daily living skills, life skills, or living skills) are tasks necessary for an individual's day-to-day functioning, and include both basic- and instrumental-level tasks.

Functional limitations and disability in these areas may range from mild to severe, as well as from short-term to lifelong.

Therapeutic intervention for ADLs is generally accepted and widely used. The goal of treatment is to improve one's ability to perform such tasks, in order to increase functional levels of independence. By including ADLs in treatment, cognitive improvements may occur by applying cognitive rehabilitation principles to the task performance. Likewise, physical deficits may be improved by applying neuromuscular rehabilitation principles to the task performance. The time to produce effect is four to five treatments, with treatments provided at three to five times per week for four to six weeks with a maximum duration of six weeks (State of Colorado 2006).

a. Basic ADL: Daily activities that tend to be repetitive, routine, and which may more readily be gained through procedural learning, such as grooming, personal hygiene, bathing/showering, toileting, dressing, feeding/eating, and basic social skills.

b. Instrumental ADL (IADL): A wide range of activities that require higher-level cognitive skills, including the ability to plan, execute, and monitor performance; evaluate information; and make sound judgments. These abilities are essential to safe, independent functioning. They may include functional communication (e.g., writing, keyboarding, appropriate use of phone), home management, child care, time management, financial management, food management, management of interpersonal relationships and social skills, avocation, driving, and higher-level mobility skills (including navigation and public transportation).

Therapeutic intervention is generally accepted to improve performance of ADLs. Procedures and techniques may include (1) task analysis to develop strategies to improve task performance, (2) guided practice and repetition to develop consistent and safe performance, (3) training in safe use of adaptive equipment, and (4) training of caregiver(s).

Interdisciplinary treatment continues until (1) functional goals/outcomes are achieved; (2) a plateau in progress is reached; (3) the individual is unable to participate in treatment due to medical, psychological, or social factors; or (4) skilled services are no longer needed.

While rate of progress will depend on the severity and complexity of the injury, effect of treatment should be noted within one month, with ongoing progress noted over a longer period, which may last up to two years or more. Treatment may be provided on an episodic basis to accommodate plateaus in the individual's progress, with suspension of treatment for periods of time to allow for practice.

Impaired cognition significantly affects the rate, degree, and manner of progress toward independence in ADLs. In addition, skills learned in one setting or circumstance may facilitate transfer of skills. All treatment to improve performance in this area must include techniques to improve cognition as well.

Standard equipment to alleviate the effects of the injury on the performance of ADLs may vary from simple to complex adaptive devices to enhance independence and safety. Certain equipment related to cognitive impairments may also be required. Equipment needs should be reassessed periodically.

Aquatic Therapy

Aquatic therapy is a well-accepted treatment that consists of the therapeutic use of aquatic immersion for therapeutic exercise to promote strengthening, core stabilization, endurance, range of motion, flexibility, body mechanics, and pain management. Aquatic therapy includes the implementation of active therapeutic procedures in a swimming or therapeutic pool. The water provides a buoyancy force that lessens the amount of force gravity applies to the body. The decreased gravity effect allows the patient to have a mechanical advantage and renders a successful trial of therapeutic exercise more likely. The therapy may be indicated for individuals who cannot tolerate active land-based or full-weight-bearing therapeutic procedures, require increased support in the presence of proprioceptive deficit, are at risk of compression fracture due to decreased bone density, have symptoms that are exacerbated in a dry environment, or would have a higher probability of meeting active therapeutic goals than in a dry environment.

The pool should be large enough to allow full-extremity range of motion and fully erect posture. Aquatic vests, belts, and other devices may be used to provide stability, balance, buoyancy, and resistance.

The time to produce effect is four to five treatments at three to five times per week for four to six weeks, with a maximum duration of eight weeks (State of Colorado 2006). A self-directed program is recommended after the supervised aquatics program has been established or, alternatively, a transition to a self-directed dry-environment exercise program.

Biofeedback

Biofeedback is a form of behavioral medicine that helps patients learn self-awareness and self-regulation skills for the purpose of gaining greater control of their physiology, such as muscle activity, brain waves, and measures of autonomic nervous system activity. There is good evidence that biofeedback and cognitive behavioral therapy are equally effective in managing chronic pain. Electronic instrumentation is used to monitor the targeted physiology and then displayed—or "fed back"—to the patient visually, aurally, or tactilely with coaching (Czosnyka and Pickard 2004).

Indications for biofeedback include individuals who are suffering from musculoskeletal injury where muscle dysfunction or other physiological indicators of excessive or prolonged stress response affects and/or delays recovery. Other applications include training to improve self-management of pain, anxiety, panic, anger or emotional distress, opioid withdrawal, insomnia/sleep disturbance, and other central and autonomic nervous-system imbalances. Biofeedback is often utilized for relaxation training.

Examples of biofeedback methods include the following:

• The electromyogram is used for self-management of pain and stress reactions involving muscle tension.
• Respiration feedback (RFB) is used for self-management of pain and stress reactions via breathing control.
• Respiratory sinus arrhythmia (RSA) is used for self-management of pain and stress reactions via synchronous control of heart rate and respiration. Respiratory sinus arrhythmia is a benign phenomenon that consists of a small rise in heart rate during inhalation, and a corresponding decrease during exhalation. This phenomenon has been observed in meditators and athletes, and is thought to be a psycho-physiological indicator of health.
• Heart rate variability (HRV) is used for self-management of stress via management of cardiac reactivity.
• Electrodermal response (EDR) is used for self-management of stress involving palmar sweating or galvanic skin response.
• The electroencephalograph (EEG, QEEG) is used for self-management of various psychological states by controlling brain waves.

The goal in biofeedback treatment is to normalize the physiology to the pre-injury status to the extent possible and involves transfer of learned skills to the workplace and daily life. Candidates for biofeedback therapy or training should be motivated to learn and practice biofeedback and self-regulation techniques. If the patient has not been previously evaluated, a psychological evaluation should be performed prior to beginning biofeedback treatment for chronic pain. The psychological evaluation may reveal cognitive difficulties, belief-system conflicts, somatic delusions, secondary gain issues, hypochondriasis, and possible biases in patient self-reports, which can affect biofeedback. Home practice of skills is often helpful for mastery and may be facilitated by the use of home training tapes.

Positive effects should be noted at around three to four sessions. Patients should be seen one to two times per week. The optimum duration is six to eight sessions, and the maximum duration of the program is ten to twelve sessions (State of Colorado 2006).

Complementary Alternative Medicine

Complementary alternative medicine is a term used to describe a broad range of treatment modalities, a number of which are generally accepted and supported by scientific research, and others that still remain outside the generally accepted practices of Western medicine.

Although complementary alternative medicine practices are diverse and too numerous to list, they can generally be classified into five domains:

1. Alternative medical systems are defined as medical practices that have developed their own systems of theory, diagnosis, and treatment and have evolved independent of and usually prior to conventional Western medicine. Some examples are traditional Chinese medicine, Ayurvedic medicine, homeopathy, and naturopathy.
2. Mind-body interventions include practices such as hypnosis, meditation, bioenergetics, and prayer.
3. Biological-based practices include herbal and dietary therapy as well as the use of nutritional supplements.
4. Body-based therapy includes practices such as yoga and Rolfing.
5. Energy-based practices include a wide range of modalities that support physical as well as spiritual and/or emotional healing. Some of the more well-known energy practices include Qi Gong, Tai Chi, Healing Touch, and Reiki. Practices such as Qi Gong and Tai Chi are taught to the patient and are based on exercises the patient can practice independently at home. Other energy-based practices such as Healing Touch and Reiki involve a practitioner-patient relationship and may provide some pain relief. Tai Chi may improve range of motion in those with rheumatoid arthritis (de Kruijk et al. 2002).

Methods used to evaluate chronic-pain patients for participation in complementary alternative medicine will differ with various approaches and with the training and experience of individual practitioners. A patient may be referred for complementary alternative medicine therapy when the patient's cultural background, religious beliefs, or personal concept of health suggests that an unconventional medical approach might assist in the patient's recovery or when the physician's experience and clinical judgment support such an approach.

Continuous Passive Movement (CPM)

Continuous Passive Movement (CPM) is a form of passive motion using specialized machinery that acts to move a joint and may also pump blood and edema fluid away from the joint and periarticular tissues. CPM is effective in preventing the development of joint stiffness if applied immediately following surgery (Dunn 2002). It should be continued until the swelling that limits motion of the joint no longer develops. ROM for the joint begins at the level of patient tolerance and is increased twice a day as tolerated.

CPM is recommended to be used up to four times a day. The optimum duration is up to three weeks postsurgery, with a maximum duration of three weeks (State of Colorado 2006).

Contrast Baths

Contrast baths are the alternating immersion of extremities in hot and cold water. Indications include edema in the sub-acute stage of healing and the need to improve peripheral circulation and decrease joint pain and stiffness. The time to produce effect is three treatments three times per week. The optimum duration is four weeks, with a maximum duration of one month (State of Colorado 2006).

Extracorporeal Shock-Wave Therapy (ESWT)

Extracorporeal Shock-Wave Therapy (ESWT) is used to increase function and decrease pain in patients with specified types of calcifying tendonitis for whom conservative therapies have failed. It is not a first-line therapy. ESWT uses acoustic impulses with a duration in microseconds focused on the target tissue. The mechanism of action is not known, but is not likely to be simply the mechanical disintegration of the calcium deposit. High-energy application of ESWT may be painful, and rare complications such as osteonecrosis of the humeral head have been reported. Dosage is established according to patient tolerance. Higher dosages are generally associated with better functional results. There is good evidence (Forsyth et al. 2001) that ESWT may improve pain and function in radiographically or sonographically defined Type I or Type II calcium deposits when conservative treatment has failed to result in adequate functional improvement, but optimal dosing has not been defined. Neither anesthesia nor conscious sedation is required, nor is it recommended for this procedure.

ESWT is indicated for patients with calcifying tendonitis who have not achieved functional goals after two to three months of active therapy. The calcium deposits must be Type I, homogenous calcification with well-defined borders, or Type II, heterogeneous with sharp border or homogenous with no defined border. The time to produce effect is three days. The optimum duration is two sessions, with a maximum duration of four sessions.

Fluidotherapy

Fluidotherapy employs a stream of dry, heated air that passes over the injured body part. The injured body part can be exercised during the application of dry heat. Indications include the need to enhance collagen extensibility before stretching, reduce muscle guarding, or reduce inflammatory response.

The time to produce effect is one to four treatments. The optimum duration is one to three times per week for four weeks, with a maximum duration of one month (State of Colorado 2006).

Infrared Therapy

Infrared therapy is a radiant form of heat application. Indications include the need to elevate the pain threshold before exercise and to alleviate muscle spasm to promote increased movement.

The time to produce effect is two to four treatments. The optimum duration is three weeks up to two months for three to five times per week (State of Colorado 2006).

Manipulation or Manipulative Treatment

Manipulative treatment is defined as the therapeutic application of manually guided forces by a therapist to improve physiologic function and/or support homeostasis that has been altered by the injury.

There is good evidence that a combination of exercise and spinal manipulation is more effective than manipulation alone in relieving chronic neck pain, and that these advantages remain for more than a year after the end of treatment (Gadkary et al. 2002).

Conversely, there is some evidence that a combination of spinal manipulation and exercise is more effective than exercise alone in reducing pain and improving function of low-back pain for one year (Naravan 2001). There is good evidence that spinal manipulation has a small superiority to other common interventions (standard medical care, physiotherapy, and exercise alone) for chronic low-back pain, making it comparable to other commonly accepted interventions for this indication (McCrory 2001).

Manipulative treatments may be applied by osteopathic physicians, chiropractors, properly trained physical or occupational therapists, or properly trained medical doctors. Some popular and useful techniques include high-velocity, low-amplitude (HVLA) treatments; muscle energy (ME); strain-counterstrain (SCS); a balanced ligamentous tension (BLT); and myofascial release (MFR). Many subsets of different techniques can be described as (a) direct—a forceful engagement of a restrictive/pathologic barrier; (b) indirect—a gentle/nonforceful disengagement of a restrictive/pathologic barrier; (c) where the patient actively assists in the treatment; and (d) where the patient relaxes, allowing the practitioner to move and balance the body tissues. When the proper diagnosis is made and coupled with the appropriate technique, manipulation has no contraindications and can be applied to all tissues of the body, including muscles, tendons, ligaments, joints, fascia, and viscera. Pretreatment assessment should be performed as part of each manipulative treatment visit to ensure that the correct diagnosis is made and the correct treatment is employed.

Contraindications to HVLA manipulation include joint instability, fractures, severe osteoporosis, infection, metastatic cancer, active inflammatory arthritides, aortic aneurysm, and signs of progressive neurologic deficits. Positive effects should be noted at around four to six treatments. Patients should be seen for one to two times per week for the first two weeks as indicated by the severity of the condition. Treatment may continue at one treatment per week for the next six weeks. The optimum duration is eight weeks. At week eight, patients should be reevaluated. Care beyond eight weeks may be indicated for certain chronic-pain patients in whom manipulation is helpful in improving function, decreasing pain, and improving quality of life. In these cases, treatment may be continued at one treatment every other week. Extended durations of care beyond what is considered "maximum" may be necessary in cases of re-injury, interrupted continuity of care, exacerbation of symptoms, and in those patients with comorbidities. Such care should be reevaluated and documented on a monthly basis. Functional gains including increased ROM must be demonstrated to justify continuing treatment (State of Colorado 2006).

Manipulation under general anesthesia involves manual manipulation of the lumbar spine in combination with the use of a general anesthetic or conscious sedation. It is intended to improve the success of manipulation when pain, muscle spasm, guarding, and fibrosis appear to be limiting its application in patients otherwise suitable for their use.

Manipulation under joint anesthesia involves manipulation of the lumbar spine in combination with a fluoroscopically guided injection of anesthetic with or without corticosteroid agents into the facet joint at the level being manipulated.

Massage

Massage is manipulation of soft tissue with broad-ranging relaxation and circulatory benefits. It may include stimulation of acupuncture points and channels (acupressure); application of suction cups; and techniques that include pressing, lifting, rubbing, or pinching of soft tissues with the practitioner's hands. Indications include edema (peripheral or hard and nonpliable edema), muscle spasm, adhesions, and the need to improve peripheral circulation and range of motion or to increase muscle relaxation and flexibility prior to exercise.

There is good evidence that massage therapy in combination with exercise reduces pain and improves function in the short term for patients with subacute low-back pain (McGarry et al. 2002).

Patients should be seen one to two times per week. The optimum duration is six weeks. The maximum duration of the program is two months (State of Colorado 2006).

Mirror Therapy—Graded Motor Imagery

Mirror Therapy—Graded Motor Imagery is accomplished through patient participation. It usually begins with limb laterality recognition, imagined motion, and mirror movements. Each phase gradually increases the number of repetitions. Therapy visits are once a week in the last phases, and the treatment is performed at home at least thirty minutes per day. There is some evidence that this therapy improves function and pain in complex regional pain syndrome (CRPS) I patients (McIntyre et al. 2003). Most of the program is accomplished through patient participation. The training period is four to eight lessons, with an optimum duration of four to six weeks with two follow-up visits (State of Colorado 2006).

Mobilization (Joint)

Mobilization is passive movement involving oscillatory motions to the vertebral segment(s). The passive mobility is performed in a graded manner

(Levels I, II, III, IV, or V), which depicts the speed and depth of joint motion during the maneuver. It may include skilled manual joint-tissue stretching. Indications include the need to improve joint play, enable segmental alignment, improve intracapsular arthrokinematics, or reduce pain associated with tissue impingement. Level V mobilization contraindications include joint instability, fractures, severe osteoporosis, infection, metastatic cancer, active inflammatory arthritides, aortic aneurysm, and signs of progressive neurologic deficits.

Positive effects should be noted at around six to nine treatments. Patients should be seen three times per week. The optimum duration is four to six weeks, with a maximum duration of six weeks (State of Colorado 2006).

Mobilization (Soft Tissue)

Mobilization of soft tissue is the skilled application of muscle energy, strain/counterstrain, myofascial release, manual trigger-point release, and manual therapy techniques designed to improve or normalize movement patterns through the reduction of soft-tissue pain and restrictions. These can be interactive, with the patient participating, or passive, with the patient relaxing and the practitioner moving the body tissues. Indications include muscle spasm around a joint, trigger points, adhesions, and neural compression. Mobilization should be accompanied by active therapy.

Positive effects should be noted at around four to nine treatments. Patients should be seen up to three times per week. The optimum duration is four to six weeks, with a maximum duration of six weeks (State of Colorado 2006).

Nerve Gliding

Nerve gliding exercises are generally accepted and consist of a series of flexion and extension movements of the hand, wrist, elbow, shoulder, and neck that produce tension and longitudinal movement along the length of the median and other nerves of the upper extremity. These exercises are based on the principle that the tissues of the peripheral nervous system are designed for movement, and that tension and glide (excursion) of nerves may have an effect on neurophysiology through alterations in vascular and axoplasmic flow. Biomechanical principles have been more thoroughly studied than clinical outcomes (Marion et al. 1997). The time to produce effect is two to four weeks with the patient performing the exercises up to five times per day (State of Colorado 2006).

Nerve gliding and upper-extremity stretching usually involve the following muscle groups: scalene, pectoralis minor, trapezius, and levator scapulae.

Endurance or strengthening of the upper extremities early in the course of therapy is not recommended, as this may exacerbate cervical or upper-extremity symptoms.

Neuromuscular Reeducation

Neuromuscular reeducation is the skilled application of exercise with manual, mechanical, or electrical facilitation to enhance strength, movement patterns, neuromuscular response, proprioception, kinesthetic sense, coordination, education of movement, balance, and posture. Indications include the need to promote neuromuscular responses through carefully timed proprioceptive stimuli, to elicit and improve motor activity in patterns similar to normal neurologically developed sequences, and to improve neuromotor response with independent control.

The time to produce effect is two to six treatments three times per week for four to eight weeks, with a maximum duration of eight weeks (State of Colorado 2006).

Orthotics

Devices and adaptive equipment may be necessary in order to reduce impairment and disability, to facilitate medical recovery, to avoid re-aggravation of the injury, and to maintain maximum medical improvement. Indications would be to provide relief of the injury, prevent further injury, and control neurological and orthopedic injuries for reduced stress during functional activities. In addition, equipment may be used to modify tasks through instruction in the use of a device or physical modification of a device.

Devices should improve safety and reduce risk of re-injury. Standard equipment to alleviate the effects of the injury on the performance of activities of daily living may vary from simple to complex adaptive devices to enhance independence and safety. Ergonomic modifications may be necessary to facilitate medical recovery, to avoid re-aggravation of the injury, and to maintain maximum medical improvement.

Fabrication/modification of orthotics, including splints, may be appropriate when there is need to normalize weight bearing, facilitate better motion response, stabilize a joint with insufficient muscle or proprioceptive/reflex competencies, protect subacute conditions as needed during movement, and correct biomechanical problems.

Orthotic/prosthetic training is the skilled instruction in the proper use of orthotic devices and/or prosthetic limbs, including stump preparation, donning and doffing limbs, instruction in wearing schedule, and orthotic/prosthetic maintenance training. Training can include activities of daily living and self-care techniques. The time to produce effect is two to six sessions when trained three times per week for two to four months (State of Colorado 2006).

Splints or adaptive equipment design, fabrication, and/or modification indications include the need to control neurological and orthopedic injuries for reduced stress during functional activities and to modify tasks through instruction in the use of a device or physical modification of a device, which reduces stress on the injury. Equipment should improve safety and reduce risk of re-injury. This includes high- and low-technology assistive options such as workplace modifications, computer interface or seating, and self-care aids.

Foot orthoses and inserts are accepted interventions for spinal disorders that are due to aggravated mechanical abnormalities, such as leg-length discrepancy, scoliosis, or lower-extremity misalignment. Shoe insoles or inserts may be effective for patients with acute low-back problems who stand for prolonged periods of time.

Lumbar support devices include backrests for chairs and car seats. Lumbar supports may provide symptomatic relief of pain and movement reduction in cases of chronic low-back problems (Airaksinen et al. 2006).

Lumbar corsets and back belts have insufficient evidence to support their use (Battie and Videman 2006). They are an accepted treatment with limited application. The injured worker should be advised of the potential harm from using a lumbar support for a period of time greater than prescribed. Harmful effects include deconditioning of the trunk musculature, skin irritation, and general discomfort (Carragee 2005).

Rigid lumbosacral bracing devices are well accepted and commonly used for postfusion, scoliosis, and vertebral fractures (Deyo and Diehl 1988).

Primary principles and objectives of the application of orthosis include (a) control of the position through the use of control forces, (b) application of corrective forces to abnormal curvatures, (c) aid in spinal stability when soft tissues or osteoligamentous structures cannot sufficiently perform their role as spinal stabilizers, and (d) restrict spinal segment movement after acute trauma or surgical procedure. In cases of traumatic cervical injury, the most important objective is the protection of the spinal cord and nerve root.

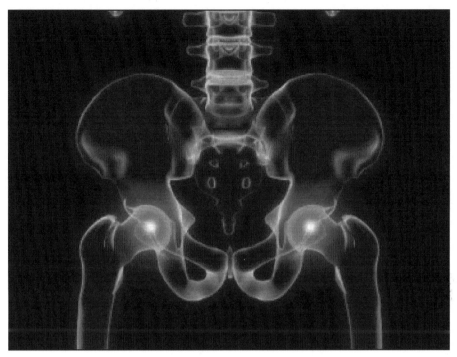

Use of cervical collars is not recommended for chronic cervical myofascial pain (Errico 2005). Special cervical orthoses and/or equipment may have a role in the rehabilitation of a cervical injury such as those injuries to a cervical nerve root resulting in upper-extremity weakness or a spinal-cord injury with some degree of paraparesis or tetraparesis. Use of such devices would be in a structured rehabilitation setting as part of a comprehensive rehabilitation program.

Soft collars are well tolerated by most patients but may not significantly restrict motion in any plane and are associated with delayed recovery. There is no evidence that their use promotes recovery from cervical sprain. In acute strain/sprain injuries, use of cervical collars may prolong disability, limit early mobilization, promote psychological dependence, and limit self-activity (Freeman et al. 1999). There is some evidence that patients encouraged to continue usual activity have less neck stiffness and headache than patients placed in cervical collars following motor vehicle crashes (Genovese 2005). Rigid collars such as a Philadelphia Orthosis are useful postsurgery or in emergency situations. These collars restrict flexion and extension motion and, to a lesser degree, lateral bending and rotation. Duration of wear postsurgery is dependent upon the surgeon and degree of cervical healing but is generally not beyond eight weeks.

Poster appliances restrict flexion and extension motion to about the same degree as a collar and restrict lateral bending and rotation to a greater degree. These are not recommended in sprain or strain injuries (Guyatt 2001).

Cervicothoracic orthoses such as Yale and sternal occipital mandibular immobilization (SOMI) braces restrict flexion and extension motion and lateral bending and rotation to a greater degree than the collar. These are not recommended in sprain or strain injuries (Hall et al. 1998).

Paraffin Bath

A paraffin bath is a superficial heating modality that uses melted paraffin (candle wax) to treat irregular surfaces such as the hand. Accepted indications include the need to enhance collagen extensibility before stretching, reduce muscle guarding, or reduce inflammatory response.

The time to produce effect is one to four treatments at one to three times per week for four weeks (State of Colorado 2006).

Patient Education

No treatment plan is complete without addressing issues of individual patient and/or group education as a means of prolonging the beneficial effects of treatment, as well as facilitating self-management of symptoms and injury prevention. Patient education is widely used, well established, and generally well accepted. Patients should take an active role in the establishment of functional outcome goals (Hansen and Helm 2003). They should be educated on their specific injury, assessment findings, and plan of treatment. Education and instruction in proper body mechanics, posture, positions to avoid, task/tool adaptation, self-care for exacerbation of symptoms, and home exercise/task adaptation should also be addressed.

In some cases, educational intervention combined with exercises may achieve results comparable to surgical intervention for patients who have undergone previous surgery (Indahl et al. 1995). There is some evidence that, for patients who had undergone previous surgery for disc herniation and continued to experience low-back pain for at least one year, educational lectures and materials in conjunction with exercise programs yield similar results, as indicated by Oswestry Disability scores for patients who had undergone posterolateral low-back fusion (Institute for Clinical Systems Improvement 2005). It should be noted that the rehabilitation program included individual and group discussions targeted toward assuring patients that participation in ordinary activities would not cause harm.

Patient education is an interactive process that provides an environment where the patient not only acquires knowledge but also gains an understanding of the application of that knowledge. Therefore, patients should be able to describe and will need to be educated on the treatment plan, indications for and potential side effects of medications, their home exercise program, expected results of treatment, tests to be performed, the reasons for such tests and their results, activity restrictions and return-to-work status, home management for exacerbated pain, procedures for seeking care for exacerbations after office hours, home self-maintenance, patient responsibility to communicate with all medical providers and the employer, patient responsibility to keep appointments, the importance of taking medications exactly as prescribed, and basic physiology related to patient's diagnosis.

Educational efforts should also extend to family and other support persons, the case manager, the insurer, and the employer to optimize the understanding of the patient and the desired outcome. Professional translators should be provided for non-English-speaking patients to assure optimum communication. All education and instruction given to the patient should be documented in the medical record.

Effects of education weaken over time; continuing patient education sessions will be required to maximize the patient's function. The effectiveness of educational efforts can be enhanced through attention to the learning style and receptivity of the patient. Written educational materials may reinforce and prolong the impact of verbal educational efforts. Overall, patient education should emphasize health and wellness, return to work, and return to a productive life.

Postural risk factors should be identified. Awkward postures of overhead reach, hyperextension or rotation of the neck, shoulder drooped or forward-flexed postures, and head-chin forward postures should be eliminated. Proper breathing techniques are also part of the treatment plan.

Postural Control

Trunk control is essential for the body to remain upright and to adjust and control movements against gravity. Postural tone and stability is evaluated by assessing the basic movement components of the upper and lower body, the coordinated trunk, extremity patterns, and the power production involved in equilibrium and protective reactions. Basic movement components of the trunk are then progressed to the linking of trunk and extremity movements in supine, sitting, and standing positions. The last level involves strength and stability for power production for activities such as walking, stair climbing, jumping, running, and throwing.

Short-Wave Diathermy

Short-wave diathermy involves the use of equipment that exposes soft tissue to a magnetic or electrical field. Benefits include enhanced collagen extensibility before stretching; reduced muscle guarding; reduced inflammatory response; and enhanced reabsorption of hemorrhage, hematoma, or edema.

The time to produce effect is two to four treatments for two to three times per week up to three weeks. The optimum duration is three to five weeks, with a maximum duration of five weeks (State of Colorado 2006).

Spinal Stabilization

The goal of this therapeutic program is to strengthen the spine in its neutral and anatomical position. The stabilization is dynamic, which allows whole-body movements while maintaining a stabilized spine. It enables the patient to move and function normally through postures and activities without creating undue vertebral stress.

The time to produce effect is four to eight treatments at three to five times per week for four to eight weeks, with a maximum duration of eight weeks (State of Colorado 2006).

Stress Loading

Stress loading is considered a reflex and sensory integration technique involving the application of a compressive load and a carry load. It is carried out in a consistent, progressive manner and integrated as part of a home program. Use of this technique may increase symptoms initially, but symptoms generally subside with program consistency. This technique is used for upper as well as lower extremities.

Positive effects should be noted at around three weeks. Patients should be seen two to three times per week. The optimum duration is four to six weeks and concurrent with an active daily home exercise program (State of Colorado 2006).

Superficial Heat and Cold Therapy

Superficial heat and cold therapy is a generally accepted treatment. Superficial heat and cold are thermal agents applied in various manners that lower or raise the body tissue temperature for the reduction of pain, inflammation, and/

or effusion resulting from injury or induced by exercise. Superficial heat therapy includes application of heat just above the surface of the skin at acupuncture points. Indications include acute pain; edema; hemorrhage; and the need to increase pain threshold, reduce muscle spasm, and promote stretching/flexibility. Cold and heat packs can be used at home as an extension of therapy in the clinic setting.

Patients should be seen two to five times per week. The optimum duration is three weeks, or intermittently as an adjunct to other therapeutic procedures for up to two months. The maximum duration of the program is two months (State of Colorado 2006).

Therapeutic Exercises and Therapeutic Activities

Therapeutic exercises and/or activities are beneficial for restoring flexibility, strength, endurance, function, and range of motion, and they can alleviate discomfort. Active therapy requires effort by the individual to complete a specific exercise or task. This form of therapy requires supervision from a therapist including verbal, visual, and/or tactile instruction. The therapist may help stabilize the patient or guide the movement pattern, but the energy required to complete the task is predominately executed by the patient. Patients should be instructed to continue active therapies at home as an extension of the treatment process in order to maintain improvement levels. Follow-up visits to reinforce and monitor progress and proper technique are recommended.

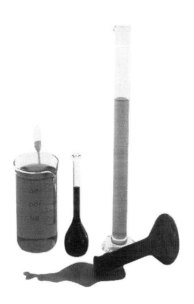

Functional activities are well-established interventions that involve the use of therapeutic activities to enhance mobility, body mechanics, employability, coordination, balance, and sensory-motor integration.

Therapeutic exercise, with or without mechanical assistance or resistance, may include isoinertial, isotonic, isometric, and isokinetic types of exercises. Benefits include cardiovascular fitness, reduced edema, improved muscle strength, improved connective-tissue strength and integrity, increased bone density, promotion of circulation to enhance soft-tissue healing, improvement of muscle recruitment, improved proprioception and coordination, increased range of motion, and promotion of normal movement patterns. Indications also include the need to promote normal gait pattern with assistive devices and/or to reduce risk of fall or loss of balance. This may include instruction in safety and proper use of assistive devices and gait instruction on uneven surfaces and steps (with or without railings). Therapeutic exercise can include complementary/alternative exercise movement as well.

The time to produce effect is two to six treatments at three to five times per week for four to eight weeks, with a maximum duration of eight weeks (State of Colorado 2006).

Traction—Manual

Manual traction is an integral component of manual manipulation or joint mobilization. Indications include decreased joint space, muscle spasm around joints, and the need for increased synovial nutrition and response. Manual traction is contraindicated in patients with tumor, infection, fracture, or fracture dislocation.

Positive effects should be noted at around one to three sessions. Patients should be seen two to three times per week (State of Colorado 2006).

Traction—Mechanical

Mechanical traction is indicated for decreased joint space, muscle spasm around joints, and the need for increased synovial nutrition and response. Traction modalities are contraindicated in patients with tumor, infections, fracture, or fracture dislocation. Non-oscillating inversion traction methods are contraindicated in patients with glaucoma or hypertension. There is some evidence (Koes et al. 2005) that mechanical traction, using specific, instrumented axial distraction technique, is not more effective than active graded therapy without mechanical traction. Therefore, mechanical traction is not recommended for chronic axial spine pain.

Positive effects should be noted at around one to three sessions up to thirty minutes each. If response is negative after three treatments, discontinue. The maximum duration is one month (State of Colorado 2006).

Vasopneumatic Devices

Vasopneumatic devices are mechanical compressive devices used in both inpatient and outpatient settings to reduce various types of edema. Indications include pitting edema, lymphedema, and venostasis. Maximum compression should not exceed minimal diastolic blood pressure. Use of a unit at home should be considered if expected treatment is greater than two weeks.

Treatment is optimally provided at three to five times per week. The optimum duration is one month (State of Colorado 2006).

Vestibular Rehabilitation

Symptoms of vestibular system dysfunction following traumatic brain injury (TBI) may be due to damage of central or peripheral structures and may include vertigo, eye-head dyscoordination affecting the ability to stabilize gaze during head movements, and imbalance affecting stability in standing or walking. Dizziness and balance disorders may or may not coexist in the same individual with TBI.

Balance is a complex motor-control task, requiring integration of sensory information, neural processing, and biomechanical factors. It is the ability to control one's center of gravity over the base of support in a given sensory environment. Balance disorders are frequently occurring symptoms following TBI. This may be due to a peripheral vestibular lesion or central vestibular lesion secondary to trauma, fracture, hemorrhage, or intracranial pressure changes.

Assessment includes evaluation of the motor system, range of motion, and sensory systems that affect the person's ability to maintain equilibrium. Movement strategies to maintain balance require functional ROM and adequate strength. Sensory information from the vestibular, visual, and somatosensory systems is a key element associated with maintenance of balance or posture, and this is integrated at the central level between the two sides of the body and three sensory systems. Central motor planning is essential for proper strategies that are then transmitted to the peripheral motor system for execution. Deficits at the central level, peripheral, motor, or sensory level will affect balance and equilibrium.

The dynamic systems model recognizes that balance and dynamic equilibrium are the result of the interaction between the individual, the functional task, and the environment. Emphasis of treatments performed by a qualified physical or occupational therapist in vestibular and balance dysfunction are head exercises for habituation of vertigo, eye-head coordination exercises for improvement of gaze stabilization, and sensorimotor retraining to remediate postural imbalances in all functional movement positions.

The time to produce effect is six to twelve weeks, with sessions initially provided daily, decreasing to one session per week after one to two weeks; individuals are expected to perform self-directed exercises twice daily at home, but may require supervision for guidance and safety. The optimum duration is six months with reevaluation; the patient may require follow-up for up to two years (State of Colorado 2006).

Wheelchair Management and Propulsion

Wheelchair management and propulsion is the instruction and training in self-propulsion and proper use of a wheelchair. This includes transferring and safety instruction. This is indicated in individuals who are not able to ambulate due to bilateral lower-extremity injuries, inability to use ambulatory assistive devices, and in cases of multiple traumas. The time to produce effect is two to six treatments for two to three times per week for two weeks (State of Colorado 2006).

Whirlpool/Hubbard Tank

The whirlpool/Hubbard tank is a generally accepted treatment in which conductive exposure to water at varied temperatures is employed to the extent that best elicits the desired effect. It generally includes massage by water propelled by a turbine or Jacuzzi jet system and has the same thermal effects as hot packs, if water temperature exceeds tissue temperature. It has the same thermal effects as cold application, if comparable temperature water is used. Indications include the need for analgesia, muscle spasm, joint stiffness, and the need to facilitate and prepare for exercise.

The time to produce effect is two to four treatments for three to five times per week. The optimum duration is three weeks as a primary treatment, or intermittently as an adjunct to other therapeutic procedures up to two months, with a maximum duration of two months (State of Colorado 2006).

Work Hardening/Work Conditioning

Early evaluation of and training in body mechanics are essential for every injured worker. Risk factors to be addressed include repetitive overhead work, lifting, and tool use. Physical factors that may be considered include use of force; repetitive work; and awkward positions requiring the use of force, vibration, and contact pressure on the nerve.

Ergonomic changes may be made to modify the hazards identified. The US Occupational Safety and Health Administration (OSHA) suggests that workers who perform overhead repetitive tasks, with or without force, take fifteen- to thirty-second breaks every ten to twenty minutes, or five-minute breaks every hour. Mini-breaks should include stretching exercises (Koes et al. 2006).

Individual characteristics, such as height or strength, affect the ideal organization of the workstation. The worksite should be adjusted to support neutral, yet natural, positions. In addition, workers should be counseled to vary tasks throughout the day whenever possible. OSHA suggests that workers who perform repetitive tasks, including keyboarding, change activities over a five-minute interval every hour. Again, mini-breaks should include stretching exercises. The following should be considered: engineering controls, e.g., mechanizing the task, and changing the tool used, or adjusting the jobsite; or administrative controls, e.g., adjusting the time an individual performs the task (Krause et al. 1997).

The following description may aid in evaluating seated work positions. The head should be in a neutral position, and if a monitor is used, there should be eighteen to twenty-four inches of viewing distance with no glare. Arms should rest naturally, with the elbow at the side and flexed to ninety degrees or slightly extended. Some individuals may prefer a wrist pad to reduce wrist extension. Wrists should be straight or minimally extended. It is generally preferable to avoid dependence on arm rests. The back must be properly supported by a chair with the back upright or leaning backwards slightly, allowing change in position with backrest adjustment. There should be good knee- and legroom, with the feet resting comfortably on the floor or footrest. Tools should be within easy reach, and twisting or bending should be avoided.

The tools should be assessed for the individual and not used universally. It is important to select the right tool for the task. In general, the person should work in the most neutral position possible and use the least force possible. For force tools, the grip should not span more than 3.5 inches, and the handle diameter should not be greater than two inches. Precision tools may require a smaller diameter. If possible, continual forearm tasks requiring supination/pronation should be avoided by using automatic tools.

Work simulation is a program where an individual completes specific work-related tasks for a particular job and geared toward return to work. Work hardening is an interdisciplinary program addressing a patient's employability and return to work. It includes a progressive increase in the number of hours per day that a patient completes work-simulation tasks until the patient can tolerate a full workday. This is accomplished by addressing the medical, psychological, behavioral, physical, functional, and vocational components of employability and return to work. A full workday is defined by the previous employment of the patient. Safe workplace practices and education of the employer and social support system regarding the person's status should be included.

Early return to work should be a prime goal in treating occupational injuries, given the poor return-to-work prognosis for an injured worker who has been out of work for more than six months. It is imperative that the patient be educated regarding the benefits of returning to work, work restrictions, and the need to follow up if problems arise. Educating the patient that pain does not need to limit activity is effective in returning patients with chronic low-back pain to work, even with minimal reported reduction of pain (Koes and van Tulder 2006). When attempting to return a patient to work after a specific injury, clear, objective restrictions of activity level should be made. An accurate job description with detailed physical duty restrictions is often necessary to assist the physician in making return-to-work recommendations.

Because a prolonged period of time off work will decrease the likelihood of return to work, the first weeks of treatment are crucial in preventing and/or reversing chronicity and the disability mindset. These programs are work-related, outcome-focused, individualized treatment programs. Objectives of the programs include improvement of cardiopulmonary and neuromusculoskeletal functions (strength, endurance, movement, flexibility, stability, and motor-control functions), patient education, and symptom relief. The goal is for patients to gain full or optimal function and return to work. The service may include the time-limited use of modalities, both active and passive, in conjunction with therapeutic exercise, functional activities, general conditioning body mechanics, and lifting techniques retraining.

These programs are usually initiated once reconditioning has been completed but may be offered at any time throughout the recovery phase. They should be initiated when imminent return of a patient to modified or full duty is not an option, but the prognosis for returning the patient to work at completion of the program is at least fair to good.

Patients should be seen two to five times per week for one to two hours per day. The optimum duration is two to four weeks, with a maximum duration of six weeks. Participation in a program beyond six weeks must be documented with respect to the need and the ability to facilitate positive symptomatic and functional gains (State of Colorado 2006).

CHAPTER 4: EVIDENCE BASED CLINICAL PRACTICE GUIDELINES

Guidelines for Low-Back Pain

The Philadelphia Panel was convened in 2001 to evaluate the strength of the scientific evidence on the efficacy of various treatment interventions for patients with low-back pain. Evidence from randomized controlled trials and observational studies was identified and synthesized using methods defined by the Cochrane Collaboration. Bias was minimized by using a systematic approach to literature research, study selection, data extraction, and data synthesis. Meta-analyses were conducted where possible (Philadelphia Panel 2001).

An expert panel was formed by inviting stakeholder professional organizations to nominate representatives. The panel developed a set of criteria for grading the strength of both the evidence and the recommendations. The Philadelphia Panel decided, based on experience that the outcomes of primary clinical importance are pain, functional status, patient global assessment, quality of life, return to work, and patient satisfaction.

The Philadelphia Panel agreed that clinical importance be defined as a clinical improvement of 15% or more relative to control. Grade A or B recommendations were required to demonstrate both clinical importance and statistical significance (grade A = good evidence to include intervention [greater than 15% relative improvement], grade B = fair evidence to include intervention, grade C = poor evidence to include or exclude intervention [less than 15% relative improvement], and ID = insufficient data). Once the methodology of gathering opinion and interpreting the evidence was defined, a feedback survey questionnaire was sent to 324 practitioners from six professional organizations to validate the recommendations. The response rate was 51%. Each positive recommendation was summarized as a one-page guideline.

The Philadelphia Panel suggested exercise (extension and strengthening) on the treatment of acute and chronic (lasting greater than twelve weeks) low-back pain were listed. There was a lack of evidence regarding efficacy for several interventions including thermotherapy, therapeutic ultrasound, massage, electrical stimulation, and mechanical traction. Further well-designed randomized controlled trials are warranted for these interventions where evidence was insufficient to make recommendations.

Guideline for Management of Back Pain After Philadelphia Review

Modality	Acute Back Pain	Chronic Back Pain
Traction	C	C
Exercise	A	A
Therapeutic Ultrasound	C	C
Neuromuscular re-education	ID	ID

Grade A= good evidence to include intervention (>15% relative improvement), grade B= fair evidence to include intervention, grade C= poor evidence to include or exclude intervention (< 15% relative improvement), ID= insufficient data.

Guidelines for Osteoarthritis

Osteoarthritis affects a large proportion of the population, and its prevalence is increasing dramatically as the populations of industrialized countries age and baby boomers enter later adulthood. In fact, the Ottawa Panel—convened to evaluate the strength of the scientific evidence on the efficacy of therapeutic exercises for patients with osteoarthritis—has estimated that the prevalence of osteoarthritis in the United States will increase from 43 million in 1997 to 60 million in 2020 (Ottawa Panel 2005). Consequently, osteoarthritis management contributes significantly to medical expenses, and the efficiency and efficacy of rehabilitation interventions bear on the direct and indirect costs of the disease.

Several systematic reviews and meta-analyses of the effectiveness of therapeutic exercise for patients with osteoarthritis have been published in scientific literature. Two meta-analyses using Cochrane Collaboration methods have been conducted for the management of patients with osteoarthritis: the effectiveness of exercise for managing patients with hip and knee osteoarthritis, and the ideal intensity of exercise for osteoarthritis management. Of three systematic reviews on the effectiveness of exercise for managing patients with osteoarthritis, one was published in a scientific journal and two were focused on the efficacy of strengthening exercises and fitness exercises. Eight other reviews exist on therapeutic exercise for arthritis. However, these reviews are out of date, were not systematic, or were not specific to osteoarthritis. Nevertheless, all of these reviews unanimously agreed that therapeutic exercise is beneficial for patients with osteoarthritis.

The trials examined two basic types of exercises. The first type was strengthening exercise, such as resistance/isometric, stretching, eccentric, and concentric exercises. These exercises were specific to different muscles. The other type was whole-body functional strengthening programs and included aerobic conditioning and general fitness. Program duration, treatment schedule for exercise intervention, and length of exercise session varied from four weeks to eighteen months for program duration, from once a week to ten times a day for treatment schedule, and from five minutes to longer duration per exercise session.

Lower-extremity strengthening versus control showed clinical benefits for pain during walking, pain ascending and descending the stairs, quadriceps femoris muscle peak torque, and timed functional tasks. Statistically significant differences were found for pain, pain while getting up from the floor, and functional status.

For lower-extremity isometric strengthening versus control, clinical benefits were found for pain getting down and up from the floor, pain while going up and down stairs, and timed functional tasks. However, benefits were not found for stiffness and functional status. Statistically significant differences were found for pain while getting down to and up from the floor.

Statistically significant differences favored concentric exercises over control for pain and functional status at eight weeks. A clinically important benefit was observed for pain but not functional status.

For concentric-eccentric versus control, clinically important benefits and statistically significant differences were observed for pain and functional status at eight weeks. Results for fifteen-meter walk, stair climbing time, and stair descending time were also significant, as were results for pain at night, pain sitting, pain rising from a chair, pain standing, and pain climbing stairs.

For whole-body functional exercise versus control, clinically important benefits were found for pain and functional status (mobility, walking, work).

The Ottawa Panel concluded that good evidence exists for the inclusion of all of the following main categories of interventions in the management of patients with osteoarthritis: strengthening exercises (grade A for pain at rest and during functional activities, ROM, grip force, level of energy, and functional status; grade C+ for quadriceps femoris muscle peak torque, specific functional activities, and timed functional activities); general physical activities, including fitness and aerobic exercises (grade A for pain during functional activities, stride length, functional status, energy level, aerobic capacity, and medication use); and manual therapy combined with exercises (grade A for pain). The recommendations related to strengthening exercises and general physical activities generally concur with all other existing guidelines.

Patients with osteoarthritis tend to adopt sedentary lifestyles. The main challenge is to find effective strategies to help these patients adopt and sustain regular physical activity habits so that they can benefit from the positive effects and avoid the negative consequences and vicious cycle of inactivity. Inactivity can lead to chronic comorbidity problems that affect joint health, functional status, and quality of life in patients with osteoarthritis. Change in lifestyle is necessary to promote sustained physical activity.

Guidelines for Therapeutic Exercise and Manual Therapy in Rheumatoid Arthritis

The purpose of this project was to create guidelines for the use of therapeutic exercises and manual therapy in the management of adult patients (greater than eighteen years of age) with a diagnosis of rheumatoid arthritis (Ottawa Panel 2005).

Rheumatoid arthritis is a systemic inflammatory disease that produces a progressive degeneration of the musculoskeletal system. A patient is said to suffer from rheumatoid arthritis if he/she meets at least four of the following seven American Rheumatism Association criteria: (1) morning stiffness for more than one hour; (2) arthritis of three or more of the following joints: right of left proximal interphalangeal joint, metacarpal joint, wrist, elbow, knee, ankle, or metatarsal joints; (3) arthritis of the hand joints (wrist, metacarpal, or proximal interphalangeal joint); (4) symmetric involvement of joints; (5) rheumatoid nodules over bony prominences, or extensor surfaces or in juxtaarticular regions; (6) positive serum rheumatoid factor; or (7) radiologic changes, including erosions or bony decalcification localized in or adjacent to the involved joints.

As one of the most prevalent chronic conditions, rheumatoid arthritis is found in approximately 1-5% of the adult population in the United States. Rheumatoid arthritis is a highly disabling disease associated with high morbidity. Even with appropriate drug therapy, up to 7% of patients are disabled to some extent five years after disease onset, and 50% are too disabled to work ten years after onset. Consequently, rheumatoid arthritis results in considerable direct costs.

The rehabilitative approach to the management of rheumatoid arthritis has nine goals: (1) to decrease pain, (2) to decrease effusion, (3) to decrease stiffness, (4) to correct or prevent joint deformity, (5) to increase range of motion, (6) to increase muscle force or decrease weakness, (7) to improve mobility and walking, (8) to increase fitness or reduce fatigue, and (9) to increase functional status (Ottawa Panel 2005).

Substantial progress has been made in the medical management of rheumatoid arthritis, but rehabilitation specialists still must provide efficient and effective interventions for their patients. The development of evidence-based clinical practice guidelines for rehabilitation of adults with rheumatoid arthritis will help patients and clinicians choose effective interventions.

The Ottawa Panel was convened to evaluate the evidence of effectiveness of ten physical rehabilitation interventions for rheumatoid arthritis. The interventions examined by the Ottawa Panel were as follows: (1) acupuncture; (2) assistive devices; (3) bed rest; (4) conservation of energy; (5) electrotherapy, including electrical stimulation, low-level laser therapy, transcutaneous electrical nerve stimulation, and therapeutic ultrasound; (6) manual therapy; (7) patient education; (8) splinting and orthotics; (9) therapeutic exercises, with an emphasis on the intensity of the exercise program; and (10) thermotherapy, including heat therapy, cryotherapy, and balneotherapy.

The primary endpoints for measurement of effectiveness were the validated and reliable outcome measures recommended by the conference on Outcome Measures for Rheumatoid Arthritis Clinical Trials and by the theoretical framework for rehabilitation application. Outcomes included organic systems and impairment, abilities and disabilities, and life habits and handicap situation. Studies were included if any one of the aforementioned outcomes was measured.

Based on previous studies in the musculoskeletal domain and on consensus, clinical improvement for all interventions studied by the Ottawa Panel was defined as 15% improvement relative to a control.

The Ottawa Panel concluded that therapeutic exercises, including specific functional strengthening and whole-body functional strengthening, are a beneficial intervention for patients with rheumatoid arthritis. Good evidence exists (grade A for pain, function, and grip force; grade B for sick leave and lower-limb muscle force; grade C+ for swollen joint) that therapeutic exercises, similar to those mentioned above, should be included as an intervention for patients with rheumatoid arthritis.

Therapeutic exercises reduce pain while improving periarticular muscle force, aerobic capacity, and joint mobility. In the presence of an inflammatory disease such as rheumatoid arthritis, a low-intensity exercise program favors the reduction of pain and an improved functional status as compared with a high-intensity program, which may exacerbate the inflammatory process and the risk of damage to the affected joints. This evidence was not reproduced in noninflammatory diseases such as osteoarthritis.

Guidelines for Electrotherapy and Thermotherapy in Rheumatoid Arthritis

The Ottawa Group, using Cochrane Collaboration methods, identified evidence-based clinical practice guidelines for the use of electrotherapy and thermotherapy interventions in the management of adult patients (greater than eighteen years of age) with a diagnosis of rheumatoid arthritis (Ottawa Panel 2005). Electrotherapeutic modalities and thermotherapy physical agents are used as part of a rehabilitation program offered mainly for pain and inflammation relief in the management of various musculoskeletal conditions. The electrotherapeutic modalities and thermal agents have been used primarily to reduce pain, effusion, and stiffness in rheumatoid arthritis. These therapeutic interventions also indirectly contribute to increased ROM, muscle force, mobility, walking ability, functional status, and physical fitness.

Low-Level Laser Therapy

Five placebo-controlled randomized trials were included in the analysis. In these trials, the low-level laser therapy treatment schedule and duration ranged from two to three sessions per week and from four to ten consecutive weeks. The dosage ranged between 2.7 and 8.1 J/cm2. A clinically important benefit was demonstrated for pain relief. Relative reductions in pain were 28% in patients with rheumatoid arthritis affecting two or more groups of joints, 25% in patients at a chronic stage, 19% in patients with rheumatoid arthritis according to established criteria, and 22% in patients with active rheumatoid arthritis. No clinically important benefit was shown for tender joints or function. The Ottawa Panel concluded that low-level laser therapy alone is beneficial for pain relief (grade A) of the foot, knee, or hand.

Low-level laser therapy irradiation positively modifies peripheral nerve activity and provides a reduction in the sensation of pain. One proposed animal model is that low-level laser therapy enhances the action of superoxide dismutase, which prevents the proliferation of prostaglandin E. This probably contributes to its anti-inflammatory and analgesic effects.

Because low-level laser therapy is rapid to administer and portable devices are available, it offers advantages for community-based services. Nevertheless, further studies are needed to determine the optimal low-level laser therapy wavelength, dosage, application techniques, and duration of intervention, and to determine long-term effects in patients with rheumatoid arthritis.

Therapeutic Ultrasound

One placebo-controlled randomized trial of therapeutic ultrasound in rheumatoid arthritis of the hand was included in the analysis. Continuous-wave ultrasound was applied in water to the dorsal and palmar aspects of the hand at 0.5 W/cm2. The therapeutic session lasted ten minutes on alternate days for three weeks for a total of ten sessions.

The Ottawa Panel found good evidence of the effects of therapeutic ultrasound for rheumatoid arthritis of the hand and posited that therapeutic ultrasound without the addition of other physical therapy interventions is effective as an intervention for rheumatoid arthritis (grade A for tender joints, grade C for swollen joints and morning stiffness).

The use of therapeutic ultrasound in rheumatoid arthritis is supported by its documented physiological effects. Both pulsed and continuous ultrasound reduce nerve conduction velocity of pain nerve fibers. Continuous ultrasound also has thermal effects that reduce muscle spasms and pain. The thermal effects also cause vasodilation, which enhances the excretion of chronically inflamed cells.

Thermotherapy
Two randomized control trials evaluated three different types of thermotherapy for rheumatoid arthritis-affected upper- and lower-extremity joints: cryotherapy, wax, and wax combined with exercise. The treatment durations ranged from five consecutive days to three times per week for four weeks. The treatment session ranged from ten to twenty minutes.

The Ottawa Panel found good evidence that thermotherapy, especially paraffin wax baths combined with exercise, benefits ROM, pain, and stiffness in the management of rheumatoid arthritis. Additionally, thermotherapy using paraffin baths combined with exercise is more effective as an adjunct therapy than it is alone. The beneficial effects of thermotherapy coincide with the physiological effects, such as facilitation of soft-tissue healing, decrease of pain through the reduction of muscle spasms, and reduction of joint stiffness.

No clinically important benefit was shown for muscle force or the pinch-function test. The Ottawa Panel found insufficient evidence on the efficacy of cryotherapy, although physiological studies have shown effects on circulatory and temperature responses, muscle spasms, and inflamed tissue.

Transcutaneous Electrical Nerve Stimulation (TENS)
Three placebo-controlled randomized trials involving TENS were included in the analysis. Three types of TENS were prescribed: low-frequency, acupuncture-like TENS; high-frequency, conventional TENS; and high- versus low-frequency TENS. The therapeutic application of TENS ranged from fifteen to twenty minutes per session and from one to fifteen consecutive sessions for up to three consecutive weeks.

The Ottawa Panel found good evidence (grade A for pain, grade C+ for global patient and power) of the effects of acupuncture-like TENS for the management of rheumatoid arthritis in the hand and wrist and recommended TENS for pain and joint swelling. However, patients with rheumatoid arthritis seem to prefer conventional TENS application compared with acupuncture-like TENS. Since both conventional and acupuncture-like TENS excite afferent fibers in the alpha-beta range, the effect is plausibly explained by the activation of intrinsic pain-suppressive systems and the concomitant release of opiates.

Guidelines for Knee Pain

Chronic knee pain is one of the most common reasons for visits to a family practitioner. Acute knee pain usually follows injury or surgery. Chronic knee pain can be related to disease such as osteoarthritis or associated with overuse or untreated injuries to muscles, ligaments, or tendons. Prospective studies show that knee pain improves with time, regardless of therapy. Nevertheless, there is a need to provide clinicians with evidence for informed decision making regarding treatment options.

The Philadelphia Panel convened to evaluate eight selected rehabilitation interventions for knee pain: (1) thermotherapy, (2) therapeutic massage, (3) therapeutic exercise, (4) electromyographic (EMG) biofeedback, (5) ultrasound, (6) TENS, (7) electrical stimulation, and (8) combined rehabilitation interventions (Philadelphia Panel 2001). Studies were eligible if they were randomized controlled trials, nonrandomized controlled clinical trials, or case-control or cohort studies that evaluated the intervention of interest in a population with knee conditions such as chondromalacia patellae, postsurgical conditions, knee osteoarthritis, and tendinitis. Rheumatoid arthritis was excluded.

The Philadelphia Panel defined outcomes of interest as functional status, pain, ability to work, patient global assessment, patient satisfaction, and quality of life. Data were analyzed for three time points post-therapy: one month, six months, and twelve months. Twenty-nine articles made the selection criteria.

The Philadelphia Panel process resulted in two clear recommendations of clinical benefit of TENS and therapeutic exercise for knee osteoarthritis. The panel concluded that traditional therapeutic exercises are beneficial for pain relief and patient global assessment in people with knee osteoarthritis (grade A for pain and patient global assessment). The feedback survey showed that 98% of the respondents agreed with the guideline. These exercises included combinations of strengthening, stretching, and functional exercises. Clinical benefit was also demonstrated for TENS for knee osteoarthritis. TENS is thought to generate neuroregulatory peripheral and central effects and modulate pain transmission.

In contrast, preoperative strengthening exercises showed no benefit on postsurgery knee function. In addition, therapeutic ultrasound did not demonstrate a clinically important benefit for osteoarthritis of the knee or for patellofemoral pain syndrome. There was insufficient data for the Philadelphia Panel to make a recommendation regarding therapeutic massage as an intervention alone for knee tendinitis, and there was poor evidence to include or exclude thermotherapy for postsurgery knee pain. The Philadelphia Panel also found there was insufficient evidence to make a recommendation regarding thermotherapy for patellofemoral pain syndrome.

Guidelines for Neck Pain

Neck pain is the second largest cause of time off from work, after low-back pain. Acute back pain is usually the result of injury or accident, most often car accidents associated with whiplash. Some studies have suggested that chronic neck pain is related to repetitive working conditions.

The most commonly prescribed intervention for the treatment of neck pain is rest, followed by analgesics. Neck pain is one of the most common conditions for referral to a therapist. Nevertheless, there is a lack of evidence for commonly used rehabilitation interventions.

The Philadelphia Panel convened to develop evidence-based clinical practice guidelines of rehabilitation interventions for nonspecific neck pain. The target users of these guidelines are physical therapists, occupational therapists, chiropractors, physiatrists, orthopedic surgeons, rheumatologists, family physicians, and neurologists. Studies were eligible if they were randomized controlled trials, nonrandomized controlled clinical trials, or case-control or cohort studies that evaluated the intervention of interest in a population of more than ten patients with nonspecific neck pain. Nonspecific neck pain was defined as pain in the neck area, with or without radiation to the extremities. The outcomes of interest were functional status, pain, ability to work, patient global improvement, patient satisfaction, and quality of life. The interventions included massage, thermal therapy, electrical stimulation, EMG biofeedback, TENS, therapeutic ultrasound, therapeutic exercises, and combinations of these treatments.

The meta-analysis showed that there is scientific evidence to support and recommend proprioceptive and traditional therapeutic exercises for chronic cervical pain. In contrast, the panel declared that there was poor evidence to include or exclude TENS for acute neck pain, based on the lack of measured effect in one randomized control trial. In addition, they found no evidence of a clinically important benefit of therapeutic ultrasound for chronic cervical syndrome. These results concur with a previous systematic review, although that review was conducted for various musculoskeletal conditions.

The main difficulty in determining the effectiveness of rehabilitative interventions is the lack of well-designed randomized controlled trials. Future research should adopt rigorous methods to detect clinically important differences with confidence.

Guidelines for Shoulder Pain

The prevalence of shoulder pain accompanied by disability is approximately 20% in the general population. Over 50% of patients diagnosed by a general practitioner to have shoulder tendinitis are referred for rehabilitation. Numerous interventions are available for the management of shoulder pain, including thermotherapy, therapeutic ultrasound, TENS, and therapeutic exercises. Among general practitioners there is a wide variety of treatment approaches. There are very few published guidelines for the management of shoulder pain. The Philadelphia Panel convened with the aim of developing the evidence-based clinical practice guidelines for shoulder pain to improve the use of appropriate interventions for this disorder (Philadelphia Panel 2001).

Eleven trials met the inclusion criteria for the analysis. Only one intervention (therapeutic ultrasound for calcified shoulder tendinitis) was shown to have a clinically important benefit. There was good agreement with this recommendation among practitioners (75%). However, ultrasound was not shown to provide clinically important benefit for nonspecific shoulder pain such as capsulitis, bursitis, or tendinitis. For several interventions and indications there was a lack of evidence regarding efficacy. Again, the main difficulty in determining the effectiveness of rehabilitation interventions is the lack of well-designed randomized controlled trials.

Guidelines for Fibromyalgia

Fibromyalgia is a rheumatologic disorder that requires the concurrent existence of chronic, widespread musculoskeletal pain and multiple sites of tenderness. Prominent symptoms include fatigue, stiffness, nonrestorative sleep patterns, and memory and cognitive difficulties. In North America, the prevalence of fibromyalgia is approximately 5% for adult women and 1.5% for adult men, with women aged fifty-five to sixty-four years most commonly affected.

The etiology and pathogenesis of fibromyalgia remain relatively unknown, severely limiting treatment success. Fewer than 50% of patients experience sufficient symptom relief. The Ottawa Methods Group convened with the aim of developing the evidence-based clinical practice guidelines for aerobic fitness exercises in the management of fibromyalgia (Brosseau et al. 2008). The Ottawa Panel subsequently convened (in 2005) to develop evidence-based clinical practice guidelines for strengthening exercises in the management of fibromyalgia.

The Ottawa Methods Group is made up of nine methodologists with extensive experience in constructing evidence-based clinical practice guidelines. The Ottawa Methods Group contacted several associations that specialize in treating fibromyalgia to nominate people with clinical experience and subsequently chose nine people in varied specialties such as rheumatology, psychology, occupational therapy, and physical therapy. The nine-member Ottawa Methods Group and the nine researchers selected joined to form the Ottawa Panel.

As noted above, the Ottawa Panel has published evidence-based clinical practice guidelines for osteoarthritis and rheumatoid arthritis, as well as stroke. The Ottawa Panel also collaborated to assess the strength of scientific evidence regarding the efficacy of therapeutic exercises for fibromyalgia. The purpose of the study was to provide effective aerobic fitness guidelines for patients, physical therapists, occupational therapists, chiropractors, rheumatologists, family physicians, kinesiologists, and other health-care professionals to assist in the overall management of fibromyalgia.

The Ottawa Panel found emerging evidence to support the use of aerobic fitness programs and strengthening exercises as part of the overall management of fibromyalgia. For aerobic exercise, most improvements found were for quality of life and pain relief. For strengthening exercises, most improvements were shown for muscle strength, quality of life, and decreases in depression. For strengthening exercises versus a control condition, statistically significant results were observed for maximal isometric knee extensor force.

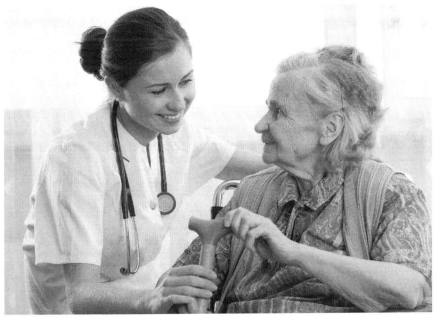

CHAPTER 5: INJECTIONS AND PHYSICIAN ADMINISTERED MODALITIES

Injections are used to temporarily weaken or paralyze muscles. They may reduce muscle pain in conditions associated with spasticity, dystonia, or other types of painful muscle spasm.

Therapeutic spinal injections may be used after initial conservative treatments—such as physical and occupational therapy, medication, manual therapy, exercise, acupuncture, etc.—have been undertaken. Therapeutic injections should be used only after imaging studies and diagnostic injections have established pathology. Injections are invasive procedures that can cause serious complications, thus clinical indications and contraindications should be closely followed.

The purpose of spinal injections is to facilitate active therapy by providing short-term relief through reduction of pain and inflammation. All patients should continue appropriate exercise with functionally directed rehabilitation. Active treatment, which patients should have had prior to injections, will frequently require a repeat of the sessions previously ordered. Injections by themselves are not likely to provide long-term relief. Rather, active rehabilitation with modified work achieves long-term relief by increasing active ROM, strength, and stability. If the first injection does not provide a diagnostic response with temporary and sustained pain relief substantiated by accepted pain scales (e.g., 80% pain reduction on visual analog scale) and improvement in function, similar injections should not be repeated (Krause et al. 1997).

For all injections (excluding trigger point), multiplanar fluoroscopic guidance during procedures is required to document technique and needle placement, and should be performed by a physician experienced in the procedure. Therapeutic injections involve the delivery of anesthetic and/or anti-inflammatory medications to the painful structure. Therapeutic injections have many potential benefits. Ideally, a therapeutic injection will reduce inflammation in a specific target area, relieve secondary muscle spasm, allow a break from pain, and support therapy directed to functional recovery. Diagnostic and therapeutic injections should be used early and selectively to establish a diagnosis and support rehabilitation. If injections are overused or used outside the context of a monitored rehabilitation program, they may be of significantly less value.

Diagnostic injections are procedures that may be used to identify pain generators or pathology. The use of injections has become progressively sophisticated. Each procedure considered has an inherent risk, and risk versus benefit should be evaluated when considering injection therapy. In addition, all injections must include sterile technique.

General contraindications include local or systemic infection, bleeding disorders, allergy to medications used, and patient refusal. Specific contraindications may apply to individual injections.

Botulinum Toxin Injections

There are several antigenic types of botulinum toxin. Botulinum toxin type B, first approved by the Food and Drug Administration in 2001, is similar pharmacologically to botulinum toxin type A. Neutralizing antibodies develop in at least 4% of patients treated with botulinum toxin type A, rendering it ineffective, but type B appears to be effective in patients who have become resistant to the type A toxin. The immune responses to botulinum toxins type A and B are not cross-reactive, allowing type B toxin to be used when type A action is blocked by antibody. Experimental work with healthy human volunteers suggests that muscle paralysis from type B toxin is not as complete or as long lasting as that resulting from type A. The duration of treatment effect of botulinum toxin type B for cervical dystonia has been estimated to be twelve to sixteen weeks. Electromyographic (EMG) needle guidance may permit more precise delivery of botulinum toxin to the target area.

Rationale for botulinum toxin as a treatment for lateral and medial epicondylitis is that it reversibly paralyzes the extensor muscles and thereby prevents repetitive microtrauma of the tendinous fibers at their origin from the osseous lateral/medial epicondyle. The unit dosage varies significantly depending on the brand used. There is good evidence that botulinum toxin A injections may provide short-term pain relief from pain due to chronic (three months or longer) lateral epicondylitis (Krause et al. 1998). However, the long-term functional benefits are unknown. There is also good evidence that botulinum toxin A injections cause weakness in finger extension and/or digit paresis. Additional complications may include allergic reaction to medications, increased risk of systemic effects in patients with motor neuropathy, or disorders of the neuromuscular junction (Krause et al. 2004).

It should not be considered a first line of treatment. Other conservative measures should be tried first. Careful botulinum toxin dosing should be used to avoid complete paresis and maintain function and return to work.

There is strong evidence that botulinum toxin A has objective and asymptomatic benefits over placebo for cervical dystonia (Linston 2000). There is some evidence (McGuirk et al. 2001) to support injections for electromyographically proven piriformis syndrome. Prior to consideration of botulinum toxin injection for piriformis syndrome, patients should have had marked (80% or better) but temporary improvement with three separate trigger-point injections. To be a candidate for botulinum toxin injection for piriformis syndrome, patients should have had symptoms return to baseline or near baseline despite an appropriate stretching program after trigger-point injections. Botulinum toxin injections of piriformis should be performed by a physician experienced in this procedure and utilize either ultrasound, fluoroscopy, or EMG needle guidance. Botulinum toxin should be followed by limb strengthening and reactivation.

Botulinum toxin injections are used for disorders that produce chronic spasticity, dystonia, or piriformis syndrome. There should be evidence (National Committee for Quality Assurance 2007) of limited range of motion prior to the injection.

There is insufficient evidence (North American Spine Society 2000) to support the use of botulinum toxin over other myofascial trigger points for longer-term pain relief, and it is likely to cause muscle weakness or atrophy if used repeatedly. Examples of such consequences include subacromial impingement, as the stabilizers of the shoulder are weakened by repeated injections into trigger points in the upper trapezii. Therefore, it is not recommended for use for other myofascial trigger points.

In terms of complications, there is good evidence (North American Spine Society 2005) that cervical botulinum toxin A injections cause transient dysphagia and neck weakness. Allergic reaction to medications, dry mouth, and vocal hoarseness may also occur. Rare systemic effects include flu-like syndrome and weakening of distant muscle. There is an increased risk of systemic effects in patients with motor neuropathy or disorders of the neuromuscular junction.

Dorsal Nerve-Root Ganglion Radiofrequency Ablation

Percutaneous radiofrequency (RF) partial lesioning of the dorsal root ganglion is a procedure intended to decrease persistent impairing radicular pain. There is some evidence (Ricci et al. 2006) that continuous RF for lumbar radicular pain does not result in improved pain and functional outcomes. Follow-up with patients who had a dorsal nerve-root ganglia procedure for failed low-back surgery revealed that two out of thirteen patients had a 50% reduction in pain and were satisfied with the procedure at two years. Fifty per cent or more of the group also reported worse sensory and motor findings. There is some evidence (Roland and Fairbank 2000) from a small study that pulsed RF, used in patients with chronic cervical radicular pain who demonstrated a 50% reduction in pain on a diagnostic block, will provide at least 50% pain relief for three months. Recurrence of pain is common after three months, with no significant effect at six months. No significant improvement in general function was documented.

Epidural Steroid Injection (ESI)

ESIs are injections of corticosteroid into the epidural space. The purpose of ESI is to reduce pain and inflammation in the acute or subacute phases of injury, restoring range of motion and thereby facilitating progress in more active treatment programs. ESI uses three approaches: transforaminal, interlaminar (midline), and caudal. The transforaminal approach is the preferred method for unilateral, single-level pathology and for postsurgical patients. There is good evidence that the transforaminal approach can deliver medication to the target tissue with few complications and can be used to identify the specific site of pathology. The interlaminar approach is the preferred approach for multilevel pathology or spinal stenosis. Caudal therapeutic injections may be used, but it is difficult to target the exact treatment area, due to diffuse distribution.

Multiplanar fluoroscopic imaging is required for all epidural steroid injections. Contrast epidurograms allow the practitioner to verify the flow of medication into the epidural space. Permanent images are required to verify needle replacement.

Cervical ESI is useful in patients with symptoms of cervical radicular pain syndromes. It has less defined usefulness in nonradicular pain. There is some evidence (Sackett and Haynes 2002) that epidural steroid injections are effective for patients with radicular pain or radiculopathy (sensory or motor loss in a specific dermatome or myotome). In one study, 53% of patients had 50% or greater relief of pain at six months with only 20% having similar relief at twelve months. There is some evidence (Speed 2004) to suggest that epidural injections are not effective for cervical axial pain; however, it is an accepted intervention. Only patients who have pain affected by activity and annular tears verified by appropriate imaging may have injections for axial pain (Waddell and Burton 2001).

There is some evidence in studies of the lumbar spine that patients who smoke or who have pain unaffected by rest or activity are less likely to have a successful outcome from ESI (Van Tulder et al. 2006). This may also apply to the cervical spine, although there are currently no studies to verify this finding. MRI or CT scans are required prior to thoracic and cervical ESI, to assure that adequate epidural space is present (Van Tulder et al. 2006).

There is some evidence that epidural steroid injections are effective for patients with radicular pain or radiculopathy (sensory or motor loss in a specific dermatome or myotome) (Waddell and Burton 2001). Up to 80% of patients with radicular pain may have initial relief. However, only 25-57% are likely to have excellent long-term relief. Although there is no evidence regarding the effectiveness of ESI for nonradicular disc herniation, it is an accepted intervention. There is some evidence that ESI is not effective for spinal stenosis without radicular findings (Waddell and Burton 2001).

Epiduroscopy and Epidural Lysis of Adhesions

Epiduroscopy and epidural lysis of adhesions is an investigational treatment of low-back pain. It involves the introduction of a fiber-optic endoscope into the epidural space via the sacral hiatus. With cephalad advancement of the endoscope under direct visualization, the epidural space is irrigated with saline. Adhesiolysis may be done mechanically with a fiber-optic endoscope. The saline irrigation is performed with or without epiduroscopy and is intended to distend the epidural space in order to obtain an adequate visual field. It is designed to produce lysis of adhesions, which are thought to produce symptoms due to traction on painful nerve roots. Saline irrigation is associated with risks of elevated pressures, which may impede blood flow and venous return, possibly causing ischemia of the cauda equina and retinal hemorrhage.

Other complications associated with instrumented lysis include catheter shearing, need for catheter surgical removal, infection (including meningitis), hematoma, and possible severe hemodynamic instability during application. Although epidural adhesions have been postulated to cause chronic low-back pain, studies have failed to find a significant correlation between the level of fibrosis and pain or difficulty functioning (Work Loss Data Institute 2011).

Intradiscal Steroid Therapy

Intradiscal steroid therapy consists of injection of a steroid preparation into the intervertebral disc under fluoroscopic guidance at the time of discography. There is good evidence that it is not effective in the treatment of suspected discogenic low-back pain (Wupperman et al. 2007).

Joint Injections

Joint injections are generally accepted, well-established procedures that can be performed as analgesic or anti-inflammatory procedures (Work Loss Data Institute 2011).

Platelet-Rich Plasma Injections

There is good evidence, in literature on lateral epicondylitis, that for patients with symptoms lasting six months or more, platelet-rich plasma injections result in better pain and functional outcomes after one year than steroid injections (Wupperman et al. 2007).

Prolotherapy

Prolotherapy, also known as sclerotherapy, consists of a series of injections of hypertonic dextrose, with or without glycerin and/or phenol, into the ligamentous structures of the low back and other joints (it has been used for "stabilization" of ankles, SI joints, etc.). Its proponents claim that the inflammatory response to the injections will recruit cytokine growth factors involved in the proliferation of connective tissue, stabilizing the ligaments of the low back or treated joints when these structures have been damaged by mechanical insults (Work Loss Data Institute 2011).

There are conflicting studies concerning the effectiveness of prolotherapy in the low back. Lasting functional improvement has not been shown. The injections are invasive, may be painful to the patient, and are not generally accepted or widely used (Van Tulder et al. 2006).

Radiofrequency Medial Branch Neurotomy/Facet Rhizotomy

This procedure is designed to denervate the facet joint by ablating the corresponding sensory medial branches. Continuous percutaneous radiofrequency is the method generally used.

There is good evidence to support radiofrequency medial branch neurotomy in the cervical spine, but benefits beyond one year are not yet established (Van Tulder et al. 2006). Evidence in the lumbar spine is conflicting; however, the procedure is generally accepted. In one study, 60% of patients maintained at least

90% pain relief at twelve months. Radiofrequency medial branch neurotomy is the procedure of choice over alcohol, phenol, or cryoablation. Precise positioning of the probe using fluoroscopic guidance is required since the maximum effective area of the device is a five-by-eight–millimeter oval.

A minority of patients with proven, significant, facetogenic low-back pain would be expected to qualify for this procedure. This procedure is not recommended for patients with multiple pain generators or involvement of more than three levels of medial branch nerves (Work Loss Data Institute 2011).

Individuals should meet all of the following criteria: pain of well-documented facet origin, unresponsive to active and/or passive therapy, and unresponsive to manual therapy. A psychosocial screening must also be performed (e.g., pain diagram, Waddell's signs, thorough psychosocial history, screening questionnaire). It is generally recommended that this procedure not be performed until three months of active therapy and manual therapy have been completed. All patients should continue appropriate exercise with functionally directed rehabilitation.

All patients should have a successful response to a diagnostic medial nerve-branch block and a separate comparative block. To be a positive diagnostic block, the patient should report a reduction of pain of 80% or greater from baseline for the length of time appropriate for the local anesthetic used. In almost all cases, this will mean a reduction of pain to one or two on the VAS ten-point scale correlated with functional improvement. The patient should also identify activities of daily living (which may include measurements of range of motion) that are impeded by their pain and can be observed to document functional improvement in the clinical setting. Ideally, these activities should be assessed throughout the observation period for function (Work Loss Data Institute 2011).

Complications can include bleeding, infection, or neural injury. The clinician must be aware of the risk of developing a localized neuritis or, rarely, a deafferentation-centralized pain syndrome as a complication of this and other neuroablative procedures.

Postprocedure therapy is active therapy, including implementation of a gentle aerobic reconditioning program (e.g., walking) and back education within the first postprocedure week, barring complications. Instruction and participation in a long-term home-based program of ROM, core strengthening, postural or neuromuscular reeducation, endurance, and stability exercises should be accomplished over a period of four to ten visits postprocedure (Work Loss Data Institute 2011).

Sacroiliac Joint Injection

Sacroiliac joint injection is a generally accepted injection of local anesthetic in an intra-articular fashion into the sacroiliac joint under radiographic guidance. It may include the use of corticosteroids. It is primarily diagnostic, to rule out sacroiliac joint dysfunction versus other pain generators. Intra-articular injection can be of value in diagnosing the pain generator. There should be documented relief from previously painful maneuvers (e.g., Patrick's test) on postinjection physical exam. These injections may be repeated if they result in increased documented functional benefit for at least six weeks and at least an 80% initial improvement in pain scales as measured by accepted pain scales. Sacroiliac joint blocks should facilitate a functionally directed rehabilitation program (Work Loss Data Institute 2011).

Shoulder-Joint Injections

Shoulder-joint injections are generally accepted, well-established procedures that can be performed as analgesic or anti-inflammatory treatments. Common shoulder-joint injections include anterior and posterior glenohumeral and acromioclavicular. Steroid injections should be used cautiously in diabetic patients. Diabetic patients should be reminded to check their blood glucose level at least daily for two weeks postinjection. There is strong evidence in literature on lateral epicondylitis that steroid injection decreases pain in the first few weeks but has a worse outcome at fifty-two weeks than physical therapy or more conservative therapy including bracing, platelet-rich plasma injections, heat or cold therapy, and change in activities (Alraksinen et al. 2006). The potential for negative long-term effects should be strongly considered. A program of physical rehabilitation in combination with judicious use of analgesic medications should be the core treatment for epicondylitis.

Soft-Tissue Injections

Soft-tissue injections include bursa and tendon insertions. Injections under significant pressure should be avoided, as the needle may be penetrating the tendon. Injection into the tendon can cause tendon degeneration, tendon breakdown, or rupture. Injections should be minimized for patients less than thirty years of age. The risk of tendon rupture should be discussed with the patient and the need for restricted duty emphasized (Work Loss Data Institute 2011).

Subacromial Injections

There is good evidence that blinded subacromial blocks are not accurate (Battie and Videman 2006). Up to a third of blinded injections may involve the cuff and are likely to cause pain. This may lead to an incorrect diagnosis when the injection is being used diagnostically (Work Loss Data Institute 2011).

Sympathetic Injections

Sympathetic injections are generally accepted, well-established procedures. They include stellate ganglion blocks and lumbar sympathetic blocks. Unfortunately, there are no high-quality randomized controlled trials in this area. It is recommended that all patients receiving therapeutic blocks participate in an appropriate exercise program that may include a functionally directed rehabilitation program.

Sympathetic Injections are indicated if greater than 50% pain relief and functional improvement is demonstrated from previous diagnostic or therapeutic blocks. Range of motion or increased strength are examples of objective gains that can be documented for most complex regional pain syndrome patients (Work Loss Data Institute 2011).

Except for Bier blocks, fluoroscopic and/or CT guidance during procedures is recommended to document technique and needle placement; an experienced physician should perform the procedure. Complications may include transient neurapraxia, nerve injury, inadvertent spinal injection, infection, venous or arterial vertebral puncture, laryngeal paralysis, respiratory arrest, vasovagal effects, as well as permanent neurologic damage.

To be effective as a treatment modality, the patient should be making measurable progress in their rehabilitation program and should be achieving an increasing or sustained duration of relief between blocks. If appropriate outcomes are not achieved, changes in treatment should be undertaken (Work Loss Data Institute 2011).

Trigger-Point Injections and Dry Needling Treatment

Trigger-point treatment can consist of dry needling or injection of local anesthetic, with or without corticosteroid, into highly localized, extremely sensitive bands of skeletal muscle fibers that produce local and referred pain when activated. Medication is injected in a four-quadrant manner in the area of maximum tenderness. Injection efficacy can be enhanced if injections are immediately followed by myofascial therapeutic interventions, such as vapocoolant spray and stretch, ischemic pressure massage (myotherapy), specific soft-tissue mobilization, and physical modalities.

There is conflicting evidence regarding the benefit of trigger-point injections. A truly blinded study comparing dry-needle treatment of trigger points is not feasible (Carragee 2005). There is no evidence that injection of medications improves the results of trigger-point injections (Deyo and Diehl 1988). Needling alone may account for some of the therapeutic response.

There is no indication for conscious sedation for patients receiving trigger-point injections. The patient must be alert to help identify the site of the injection.

Trigger-point injections may be used to relieve myofascial pain and facilitate active therapy and stretching of the affected areas. They are to be used as an adjunctive treatment in combination with other treatment modalities such as functional restoration programs. Trigger-point injections should be utilized primarily for the purpose of facilitating functional progress. Patients should continue in an aggressive aerobic and stretching therapeutic exercise program as tolerated throughout the time period they are undergoing intensive myofascial interventions. Myofascial pain is often associated with other underlying structural problems and any abnormalities must be ruled out prior to injection.

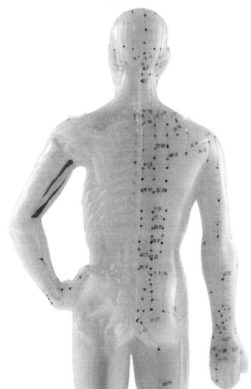

Trigger-point injections are indicated in those patients where well-circumscribed trigger points have been consistently observed, demonstrating a local twitch response, characteristic radiation of pain pattern, and local autonomic reaction, such as persistent hyperemia following palpation. Generally, these injections are not necessary unless consistently observed trigger points are not responding to specific, noninvasive, myofascial interventions within approximately a six-week timeframe (Work Loss Data Institute 2011).

Potential but rare complications of trigger-point injections include infection, pneumothorax, anaphylaxis, neurapraxia, and neuropathy. If corticosteroids are injected in addition to local anesthetic, there is a risk of local myopathy developing. Severe pain on injection suggests the possibility of an intraneural injection, and the needle should be immediately repositioned.

Viscosupplementation/Intracapsular Acid Salts

Viscosupplementation, or intracapsular acid salts, involves the injection of hyaluronic acid and its derivatives into the glenohumeral joint space. Hyaluronic acid is secreted into the joint space by the healthy synovium and has functions of lubrication and cartilage protection. Its use in the shoulder is not supported by scientific evidence at this time (Errico 2005).

Viscosupplementation is an accepted form of treatment for osteoarthritis or degenerative changes in the knee joint. While there is good scientific evidence to support their use, studies have not included patients with severe (Grade 4) degenerative changes. It is recommended that these injections be considered a therapeutic alternative in patients who have failed nonpharmacological and analgesic treatment, particularly if NSAID treatment is contraindicated or surgery is not an option (Work Loss Data Institute 2011).

Zygapophyseal (Facet) Injection

This treatment is generally accepted and involves an intra-articular or pericapsular injection of local anesthetic and corticosteroid. There is conflicting evidence to support long-term therapeutic effects using facet injections. There is no justification for a combined facet and medial branch block (Freeman et al. 1999).

In patients with pain suspected to be facet in origin based on exam findings and affecting activity, patients who have refused a rhizotomy, or patients who have facet findings with a thoracic component, facet injections may be occasionally useful in facilitating a functionally directed rehabilitation program and to aid in identifying pain generators. Patients with recurrent pain should be evaluated with more definitive diagnostic injections, such as medial nerve branch injections, to determine the need for a rhizotomy. Because facet injections are not likely to produce long-term benefit by themselves and are not the most accurate diagnostic tool, they should not be performed at more than two levels.

Facet injections may be repeated if they result in increased documented functional benefit for at least four to six weeks and at least an 80% initial improvement in pain scales as measured by accepted pain scales (Work Loss Data Institute 2011).

CHAPTER 6: COMMON MEDICATIONS

There is no single formula for pharmacological treatment of patients with chronic nonmalignant pain. A thorough medication history, including use of alternative and over-the-counter medications, should be performed at the time of the initial visit and updated periodically. The medication history may consist of evaluating patient refill records through pharmacies to determine if the patient is appropriately taking their prescribed regimen. Appropriate application of pharmacological agents depends on the patient's age, past history (including history of substance abuse), drug allergies, and the nature of all medical problems.

It is incumbent upon the health-care provider to thoroughly understand pharmacological principles when dealing with the different drug families, their respective side effects, drug interactions, bioavailability profiles, and primary reason for each medication's usage. Patients should be aware that medications alone are unlikely to provide complete pain relief. In addition to pain relief, a primary goal of drug treatment is to improve the patient's function as measured behaviorally. In addition to taking medications, continuing participation in exercise programs and using self-management techniques such as biofeedback, cognitive behavioral therapy, and other individualized physical and psychological practices are essential elements for successful chronic pain management.

Control of chronic nonmalignant pain is expected to involve the use of medication. Strategies for pharmacological control of pain cannot be precisely specified in advance. Rather, drug treatment requires close monitoring of the patient's response to therapy, flexibility on the part of the prescriber, and a willingness to change treatment when circumstances change. Many of the drugs discussed in the medication section were licensed for indications other than analgesia, but are effective in the control of some types of chronic pain.

All medications should be given an appropriate trial in order to test for therapeutic effect. The length of an appropriate trial varies widely depending on the individual drug. Certain medications may take several months to determine the efficacy, while others require only a few doses.

Acetaminophen

Acetaminophen is an effective analgesic with antipyretic but not anti-inflammatory activity. Acetaminophen is generally well tolerated, causes little or no gastrointestinal irritation, and is not associated with ulcer formation. Acetaminophen has been associated with liver toxicity in overdose situations or in chronic alcohol use. Long-term use of this substance for three days per week or more may be associated with rebound pain upon cessation.

Bisphosphonates

Bisphosphonates are potent inhibitors of bone resorption. There is good evidence that their use effectively decreases pain and some evidence they increase joint motion in patients with complex regional pain syndrome (Guyatt 2001). One study used alendronate 40 mg orally for eight weeks and another used IV clodronate 300 mg daily for ten days. The FDA has not approved use for this indication. It should not be used in those with severe renal dysfunction. Osteonecrosis of the jaw has been reported, and there may be an association with atypical subtrochanter femoral fractures, especially with long term use. The recommended dosage and time period for treatment are not clear (Hall et al. 1998).

Calcitonin

Calcitonin has been described in two low-quality studies and was not shown to benefit CRPS patients. It was thought to provide analgesic properties through the release of b-endorphin and the inhibition of bone resorption. It is not approved by the FDA for use with CRPS (Indahl et al. 1995).

Glucosamine

There is good evidence that glucosamine does not improve pain-related disability in those with chronic low-back pain and degenerative changes on radiologic studies, and therefore it is not recommended for chronic lower-spinal or non-joint pain (Hansen, and Helm 2003).

Muscle Relaxants, Skeletal Muscle Relaxants

Muscle relaxants are appropriate for muscle spasm with pain. There is strong evidence that muscle relaxants are effective for short-term pain relief in acute low-back pain. Similar effects can be expected for cervical pain. Side effects include drowsiness or dizziness, and benzodiazepines may be habit-forming (Institute for Clinical Systems Improvement 2005).

Skeletal muscle relaxants are most useful for acute musculoskeletal injury or exacerbation of injury. Chronic use of benzodiazepines or any muscle relaxant is not recommended due to their habit-forming potential, seizure risk following abrupt withdrawal, and documented contribution to deaths of patients on chronic opioids due to respiratory depression. Baclofen may be effective due to stimulation of gamma aminobutyric acid (GABA) receptors. Cyclobenzaprine can be used for acute or exacerbated chronic pain associated with muscle spasm. Central acting muscle relaxants such as Metaxalone can be used for muscle spasm.

Narcotics

Narcotics should be primarily reserved for the treatment of severe pain. Adverse effects include respiratory depression, the development of physical and psychological dependence, and impaired alertness. Narcotic medications should be prescribed with strict time, quantity, and duration guidelines, and with definitive cessation parameters. Pain is subjective in nature and should be evaluated using a scale to rate effectiveness of the narcotic prescribed (Institute for Clinical Systems Improvement 2005).

Nonsteroidal Anti-Inflammatory Drugs (NSAIDs)

Nonsteroidal anti-inflammatory drugs (NSAIDs) are useful for pain and inflammation. In mild cases, they may be the only drugs required for analgesia. The FDA advises that many NSAIDs may cause an increased risk of serious cardiovascular thrombotic events, myocardial infarction, and stroke, which can be fatal. Naproxen sodium does not appear to be associated with increased risk of vascular events. Administration of proton-pump inhibitors, histamine-2 blockers, or prostaglandin-analog misoprostol along with these NSAIDs may reduce the risk of duodenal and gastric ulceration but do not affect possible cardiovascular complications. NSAIDs are associated with abnormal renal function, including renal failure, as well as abnormal liver function. Serious gastrointestinal toxicity, such as bleeding, perforation, and ulceration can occur at any time, with or without warning symptoms in patients treated with traditional NSAIDs (Institute for Clinical Systems Improvement 2005).

Selective cyclo-oxygenase-2 (COX-2) inhibitors are more recent NSAIDs and have less gastrointestinal toxicity and no platelet effects. COX-2 inhibitors can worsen renal function in patients with renal insufficiency, thus renal function may need monitoring (Institute for Clinical Systems Improvement 2005).

Opioids

Opioids are the most powerful analgesics. Their use in acute pain and moderate to severe cancer pain is well accepted. Opioids include some of the oldest and most effective drugs used to control severe pain. In most cases, analgesic treatment should begin with acetaminophen, aspirin, and NSAIDs. While maximum efficacy is modest, they may reduce pain sufficiently to permit adequate function. Most studies show that only around 50% of patients tolerate opioid side effects and receive an acceptable level of pain relief (Jenner and Barry 1995). Common side effects are drowsiness, constipation, nausea, and possible testosterone decrease with longer-term use.

Steroids, Oral

Inflammation is thought to be one of the first physiological changes in complex regional pain syndrome; therefore, strong anti-inflammatories should provide some relief, especially if prescribed early. There is some evidence to support oral steroid use early in the course of CRPS (Jordan et al. 2011). The strongest study was performed on patients with CRPS of the shoulder and hand following a stroke. Forty milligrams of prednisone were given for fourteen days and then tapered by ten milligrams per week while physical therapy was provided. Side effects in some patients include mood changes, fluid retention, hyperglycemia, gastric irritation and ulcers, and aseptic necrosis (Koes et al. 2001).

Topical Agents

Topical medications, such as lidocaine and capsaicin, may be an alternative treatment for neuropathic disorders and are an acceptable form of treatment in selected patients. Side effects include localized skin reactions, depending on the medication agent used. Formulations of capsaicin have been approved by the FDA for management of pain associated with post-herpetic neuralgia. Capsaicin offers a safe and effective alternative to systemic NSAID therapy. Although it is quite safe, effective use of capsaicin is limited by the local stinging or burning sensation that typically dissipates with regular use, usually after the first seven to ten days of treatment. Patients should be advised to apply the cream on the affected area with a plastic glove or cotton applicator and to avoid inadvertent contact with eyes and mucous membranes. There is good evidence that low-dose capsaicin (0.075%) applied four times per day will decrease pain up to 50% (Koes and van Tulder 2005). There is also good evidence that a high-dose (8%) capsaicin patch applied for sixty minutes can decrease post-herpetic neuralgic pain for three months and thus may be useful in other chronic neuropathies (Koes et al. 2006).

Combinations of ketamine and amitriptyline have been proposed as an alternative treatment for neuropathic disorders, including CRPS. A study using a 10% concentration showed no signs of systemic absorption.

Topical salicylates and nonsalicylates have been shown to be effective in relieving pain in acute musculoskeletal conditions and single joint osteoarthritis. There is good evidence that diclofenac gel reduces pain and improves function in mild to moderate hand osteoarthritis (Koes and van Tulder 2006). Formulations of diclofenac gel have been approved by the FDA for acute pain due to minor strains, pains, and contusions, and for relief of pain due to osteoarthritis of the joints amenable to topical treatment, such as those of the knees and hands. Topical salicylates and nonsalicylates have been shown to be effective in relieving pain in acute and chronic musculoskeletal conditions. Topical salicylates and nonsalicylates achieve tissue levels that are potentially therapeutic, at least with regard to COX inhibition.

There is some evidence that topical ketoprofen patches are more effective than placebo in reducing the pain of upper-extremity tendinitis; however, the need for continuous skin application may limit overall use (Krause et al. 1997). Other than local skin reactions, the side effects of therapy are minimal, although not nonexistent, and the usual contraindications to use of these compounds should be considered. Local skin reactions are rare, and systemic effects were even less common. Their use in patients receiving warfarin therapy may result in alterations in bleeding time. Overall, the low level of systemic absorption can be advantageous, allowing the topical use of these medications when systemic administration is relatively contraindicated, such as in patients with hypertension, cardiac failure, or renal insufficiency. Hepatic changes have been documented with topical NSAID use, and therefore monitoring of liver enzymes is recommended (Institute for Clinical Systems Improvement 2005).

Topical drug delivery may be an alternative treatment for localized musculoskeletal disorders. All topical agents must be used with strict instructions for application as well as the maximum number of applications per day to obtain the desired benefit and avoid potential toxicity. As with all medications, patient selection must be rigorous to select those patients with the highest probability of compliance.

Tramadol

Tramadol is useful in relief of pain and has been shown to provide pain relief equivalent to that of commonly prescribed NSAIDs. Although Tramadol may cause impaired alertness, it is generally well tolerated and does not cause gastrointestinal ulceration or exacerbate hypertension or congestive heart failure.

Tramadol should be used cautiously in patients who have a history of seizures or who are taking medication that may lower the seizure threshold, such as monoamine oxidase (MAO) inhibitors, selective serotonin reuptake inhibitors (SSRIs), and tricyclic antidepressants. This medication has physically addictive properties, and withdrawal may follow abrupt discontinuation. It is not recommended for those with prior opioid addiction (Institute for Clinical Systems Improvement 2005).

Vitamin B6

Randomized trials on nonsurgical treatment for carpal tunnel syndrome have demonstrated conflicting results. Higher doses may result in development of a toxic peripheral neuropathy. In the absence of definitive literature showing a beneficial effect, use of Vitamin B6 cannot be recommended (Krause et al. 1997).

Vitamin C

There is some evidence that 500mg of Vitamin C, taken for fifty days after a wrist fracture, may help to prevent complex regional pain syndrome (Krause et al. 1998). It may be useful to prescribe Vitamin C to patients who have had or currently have CRPS if they suffer a fracture in order to prevent exacerbation of the syndrome.

Numerous guidelines recommend therapeutic modalities for the management of musculoskeletal conditions; however, recommendations are lacking concerning the specific adjunct modalities to employ. Evidence-based clinical practice guidelines have been developed to address this issue. Many are purported—without documentation—to be effective nonsurgical options for the treatment of pain. Keeping that in mind, any prescription should include the diagnosis; type, frequency, and duration of the prescribed therapy; therapeutic goals; and safety precautions. Clearly, future research should include randomized, placebo-controlled trials to evaluate the effectiveness of adjunct modalities in the treatment of neurologic and musculoskeletal conditions.

REFERENCES

Airaksinen, O., Brox, J.L., Cedraschi, C., Hildebrandt, J., Klaber-Moffett, J. Kovacs, F...Zanoli, G. "Chapter 4: European Guidelines for the Management of Chronic Nonspecific Low Back Pain." Supplement, European Spine Journal 15, no. S2 (2006): S192-300. doi:10.1007/s00586-006-1072-1.

Alexander, L.D., D.R. Gilman, D.R. Brown, J.L. Brown, and P.E. Houghton. "Exposure to Low Amounts of Ultrasound Energy Does Not Improve Soft Tissue Shoulder Pathology: A Systematic Review." Physical Therapy 90, no. 1 (2010): 14-25. doi:10.2522/ptj.20080272.

Artho, P.A., J.G. Thyne, B.P. Warring, C.D. Willis, J.M. Brismee, and N.S. Latman. "A Calibration Study of Therapeutic Ultrasound Units." Physical Therapy 82, no. 3 (2002): 257-63. http://ptjournal.apta.org/content/82/3/257.long.

Baker, K.G., V.J. Robertson, and F.A. Duck. "A Review of Therapeutic Ultrasound Biophysical Effects." Physical Therapy 81, no. 7 (2001): 1351-58. http://ptjournal.apta.org/content/81/7/1351.long.

Battie, M.C., and T. Videman. "Lumbar Disc Degeneration: Epidemiology and Genetics." Supplement, Journal of Bone and Joint Surgery 88, no. S2 (2006): 3-9.

Beattie, P.F., R.M. Nelson, L.A. Michener, J. Cammarata, and J. Donley. "Outcomes after a Prone Lumbar Traction Protocol for Patients with Activity-Limiting Low Back Pain: A Prospective Case Series Study." Archives of Physical Medicine and Rehabilitation 89, no. 2 (2008): 269-74. doi:10.1016/j.apmr.2007.06.778.

Bell, A.L., and J. Cavorsi. "Noncontact Ultrasound Therapy for Adjunctive Treatment of Nonhealing Wounds: Retrospective Analysis." Physical Therapy 89, no. 1 (2008): 103. http://ptjournal.apta.org/content/88/12/1517.long.

Bigos, S., O. Bowyer, G. Braen, K. Brown, R. Devo, and S. Haldeman. "Acute Low Back Problems in Adults." Clinical Practice Guideline No. 14. AHCPR Publication No. 95-0642. (Rockville, MD, Agency for Healthcare Policy and Research, Public Health Service, US Department of Health and Human Services, December 1994). http://d4c2.com/d4c2-000038.htm.

Borman, P., D. Keskin, and H. Bodhur. "The Efficacy of Lumbar Traction in the Management of Patients with Low Back Pain." Rheumatology International 23, no. 2 (2003): 82-86. http://link.springer.com/article/10.1007%2Fs00296-002-0249-0.

Brosseau, L., Robinson, V., Wells, G., Debie, R., Garn, A., Harman, K... Tugwell, P. "Low Level Laser Therapy (Classes I, II And III) for Treating Rheumatoid Arthritis." Cochrane Database System Reviews 19, no. 4 (2005). doi:10.1002/14651858.CD002049.pub2.

Brosseau, L., Wells, G.A., Tugwell, P., Egan, M., Wilson, K.G., Dubouloz, C.J....Veilleux, L. "Ottawa Panel Evidence-Based Clinical Practice Guidelines for Aerobic Fitness Exercises in the Management of Fibromyalgia:

Part 1." Physical Therapy 88, no. 7 (2008): 857-71. doi:10.2522/ ptj.20070200.

Brosseau, L., Wells, G.A., Tugwell, P., Egan, M., Wilson, K.G., Dubouloz, C.J....Veilleux, L. (2008). "Ottawa Panel Evidence-Based Clinical Practice Guidelines for Strengthening Exercises in the Management of Fibromyalgia: Part 2." Physical Therapy 88, no. 7 (2008): 873-60. doi:10.2522/ ptj.20070115.

Bulger, E.M., A.B. Nathens, F.P. Rivara, M. Moore, E.J. MacKenzie, and G.J. Jurkovich. "Management of Severe Head Injury: Institutional Variations in Care and Effect on Outcome." Critical Care Medicine 30, no. 8 (2002): 1870-76. http://journals.lww.com/ccmjournal/pages/articleviewer.aspx?year= 2002&issue=08000&article=00033&type=abstract.

Busse, J.W., M. Bhandari, A.V. Kulkami, and E Tunks. "The Effect of Low-Intensity Ultrasound Therapy on Time to Fracture Healing: A Meta-Analysis." Canadian Medical Association Journal 166, no. 4 (2002): 437-41. http://www.ncbi.nlm.nih.gov/pmc/articles/PMC99352/.

Carragee, E. J. "Persistent Low Back Pain." New England Journal of Medicine 352, no. 18 (2005): 1891-98. http://www.nejm.org/doi/full/10.1056/ NEJMcp042054.

Ciccone, C.D. "Evidence in Practice: Answers Are within Your Reach." Physical Therapy 84, no. 1 (2004): 6-7. http://ptjournal.apta.org/content/84/1/6. extract?sid=7ab3df3c-23a8-403a-a324-0bd5855d91d9.

Claes, L., and B. Willie. "The Enhancement of Bone Regeneration by Ultrasound." Progress in Biophysics and Molecular Biology 93, nos. 1–3 (2007): 384-98. doi:10.1016/j.pbiomolbio.2006.07.021.

Clarke, J.A., M.W. van Tulder, S.E. Blomberg, H.C. de Vet, G.J. van der Heijden, G. Bronfort, and L.M. Bouter. "Traction for Low Back Pain with or without Sciatica." Cochrane Database of Systematic Reviews 18, no. 2 (2007). http://onlinelibrary.wiley.com/doi/10.1002/14651858.CD003010. pub4/full.

Clifton, G.L. "Is Keeping Cool Still Hot? An Update on Hypothermia in Brain Injury." Current Opinion in Critical Care 10, no. 2 (2004): 116-19. http:// journals.lww.com/co-criticalcare/pages/articleviewer.aspx?year=2004&issue= 04000&article=00007&type=abstract.

Clifton, G.L., Miller, E.R., Choi, S.C., Levin, H.S., McCauley, S., Smith, K.R.... Schwartz, M. "Lack of Effect of Induction of Hypothermia after Acute Brain Injury." New England Journal of Medicine 344, no. 8 (2001): 556-63. http:// www.nejm.org/doi/full/10.1056/NEJM200102223440803.

College of Physiotherapists of Ontario. Clinical Guidelines on Spinal Manipulation. Ontario, Canada: 1998.

Czosnyka, M., and J.D. Pickard. "Monitoring and Interpretation of Intracranial Pressure." Journal of Neurology, Neurosurgery and Psychiatry 75, no. 6 (2004): 813-21. http://www.ncbi.nlm.nih.gov/pmc/articles/PMC1739058/.

de Kruijk, J.R., P. Leffers, S. Meerhoof, J. Rutten and N. Twijnstra.

"Effectiveness of Bed Rest after Mild Traumatic Brain Injury: A Randomized Trial of No versus Six Days of Bed Rest. Journal of Neurology, Neurosurgery and Psychiatry 73, no. 2 (2002): 167-72. http://www.ncbi.nlm.nih.gov/pmc/articles/PMC1737969/.

Deyo, R.A., and A.K. Diehl. "Cancer as a Cause of Back Pain: Frequency, Clinical Presentation, and Diagnostic Strategies." Journal of General Internal Medicine 3, no. 3 (1988): 230-38.

Draper, D.O., J.C. Castel, and D. Castel. "Rate of Temperature Increase in Human Muscle During 1 MHz and 3 MHz Continuous Ultrasound." Journal of Orthopaedic and Sports Physical Therapy 22, no. 4 (1995): 142-50.

Gebauer, D., E. Mayr, E. Orthner, and J.P. Ryaby. "Low-Intensity Pulsed Ultrasound: Effects on Nonunions." Ultrasound in Medicine and Biology 31, no. 10 (2005): 1391-1402. http://www.umbjournal.org/article/S0301-5629(05)00249-8/abstract.

Dunn, L.T. "Raised intracranial pressure." Supplement, Journal of Neurology, Neurosurgery and Psychiatry 73, no. S1 (2002): i23-7. http://www.ncbi.nlm.nih.gov/pmc/articles/PMC1765599/.

Errico, T.J. "Syntegration: A 'More Complete' Knowledge-Based Approach to the Practice of Medicine—North American Spine Society Presidential Address, Chicago, IL." The Spine Journal 5, no. 1 (2005): 6-12.

Forsyth, R., P. Baxter, and T. Elliott. "Routine Intracranial Pressure Monitoring in Acute Coma." Cochrane Database of Systematic Reviews 3 (2001). doi:10.1002/14651858.CD002043.

Freeman, M.D., A.C. Croft, A.M. Rossignol, D.S. Weaver, and Reiser. "A Review and Methodological Critique of the Literature Refuting Whiplash Syndrome." Spine 23, no. 1 (1999): 86-96.

Fung, D.T., G.Y. Ng, M.C. Leung, and D.K. Tay. "Therapeutic Low Energy Laser Improves the Mechanical Strength of Repairing Medial Collateral Ligament." Lasers in Surgical Medicine 31, no. 2 (2002): 91-96. doi:10.1002/lsm.10083.

Gadkary, C.S., P. Alderson, and D.F. Signorini. "Therapeutic Hypothermia for Head Injury." Cochrane Database of Systematic Reviews 1 (2002). doi:10.1002/14651858.CD001048.

Genovese, E. "Acupuncture—Medical Literature Analysis and Recommendations: ACOEM's Practice Guideline." APG Insights 2–10 (Winter 2005).

Gregory, C.M., and C.S. Bickel. "Recruitment Patterns in Human Skeletal Muscle during Electrical Stimulation." Physical Therapy 85, no. 4 (2005): 358-64. http://ptjournal.apta.org/content/85/4/358.long.

Gursel, Y.K., Y. Ulus, A. Bilgic, G. Dincer, and G.J. van der Heijden. "Adding Ultrasound in the Management of Soft Tissue Disorders of the Shoulder: A Randomized Placebo-Controlled Trial." Physical Therapy 84, no. 4 (2004): 336-43. http://ptjournal.apta.org/content/84/4/336.long.

Guyatt, G. Users' Guide to the Medical Literature: A Manual for Evidence-

Based Clinical Practice. New York, NY: American Medical Association, 2001.

Hadjiargyrou, M., K. McLeod, J.P. Ryaby, and C. Rubin. "Enhancement of Fracture Healing by Low Intensity Ultrasound." Supplement, Clinical Orthopaedics and Related Research 355 (1998): S216-19.

Hall, H., G. McIntosh, L. Wilson, and T. Melles. "Spontaneous Onset of Back Pain." Clinical Journal of Pain 14, no. 2 (1998): 129-33.

Hansen, H.C., and S. Helm II. "Sacroiliac Joint Pain and Dysfunction." Pain Physician 6, no. 2 (2003): 179-89. http://www.painphysicianjournal.com/linkout_vw.php?issn=1533-3159&vol=6&page=179.

Heckman, J.D., J.P. Ryaby, J. McCabe, J.J. Frey, and R.F. Kilcoyne. "Acceleration of Tibial Fracture-Healing by Noninvasive, Low-Intensity Pulsed Ultrasound." Journal of Bone and Joint Surgery, American Volume 76, no. 1 (1994): 26-34.

Hecox, B., T. Andemicael Mehreteab, and J. Weisberg. Physical Agents: A Comprehensive Text for Physical Therapists. Norwalk, CT: Appleton & Lange, 1994.

Hekkenberg, R.T., K. Beissner, B. Zegiri, R.A. Bezemer, and M. Hodnett. "Validated Ultrasonic Power Measurements up to 20 W." Ultrasound in Medicine and Biology 27, no. 3 (2001): 427-38. http://www.umbjournal.org/article/S0301-5629(00)00344-6/abstract.

Hochberg, M.C., Altman, R.D., Brandt, K.D., Clark, B.M., Dieppe, P.A., Griffin, M.R...Schnitzer, T.J. "Guidelines for the Medical Management of Osteoarthritis, Part II: Osteoarthritis of the Knee." Arthritis and Rheumatism 38, no. 11 (1995): 1541-46.

Indahl, A., L. Velund, and O. Reikeraas. "Good Prognosis for Low Back Pain When Left Untampered: A Randomized Clinical Trial." Spine 20, no. 4 (1995): 473-77.

Institute for Clinical Systems Improvement. Adult Low Back Pain. Bloomington, MN: Institute for Clinical Systems Improvement, 2005.

Jenner, J.R., and M. Barry. "ABC of Rheumatology: Low Back Pain." BMJ 310, no. 6984 (1995): 929-32. http://www.ncbi.nlm.nih.gov/pmc/articles/PMC2549345/.

Johansson, K.M., L.E. Adolfsson, and M.O. Foldevi. "Effects of Acupuncture versus Ultrasound in Patients with Impingement Syndrome: Randomized Clinical Trial." Physical Therapy 85, no. 6 (2005): 490-501. http://ptjournal.apta.org/content/85/6/490.long.

Jordan, J., K. Konstantinou, and J. O'Dowd. "Herniated Lumbar Disc." Clinical Evidence 28 (2011): pii:1118. http://www.ncbi.nlm.nih.gov/pubmed/21711958.

Khan, Y. and C.T. Laurencin. "Fracture Repair with Ultrasound: Clinical and Cell-Based Evaluation." Supplement, The Journal of Bone and Joint Surgery, American Volume 90, no. S1 (2008): 138-44. doi:10.2106/JBJS.G.01218.

Klucinec, B., M. Scheidler, C. Denegar, E. Dornholdt, and S. Burgess.

"Effectiveness of Wound Care Products in the Transmission of Acoustic Energy." Physical Therapy 80, no. 5 (2000): 469-76. http://ptjournal.apta.org/content/80/5/469.long.

Koes, B., and M. van Tulder. "Low Back Pain (Acute)." Clinical Evidence 14 (2005): 1446-57.

Koes, B., and M. van Tulder. "Low Back Pain (Chronic)." Clinical Evidence 15 (2006): 1634-53.

Koes, B.W., M.W. van Tulder, and S. Thomas. "Diagnosis and Treatment of Low Back Pain." BMJ 332, no. 7555 (2006): 1430-34. http://www.bmj.com/content/332/7555/1430?view=long&pmid=16777886.

Koes, B.W., M.W. van Tulder, R. Ostelo, B.A. Kim, and G. Waddell. "Clinical Guidelines for the Management of Low Back Pain in Primary Care: An International Comparison." Spine 26, no. 22 (2001): 2504-14.

Krause, N., D.R. Ragland, J.M. Fisher, and S.L. Syme. "Psychosocial Job Factors, Physical Workload and Incidence of Work-Related Spinal Injury: A 5-Year Prospective Study of Urban Transit Operators." Spine 23, no. 23 (1998): 2507-16. http://journals.lww.com/spinejournal/pages/articleviewer.aspx?year=1998&issue=12010&article=00005&type=abstract.

Krause, N., D.R. Ragland, B.A. Greiner, J.M. Fisher, B.L. Holman, and S. Selvin. "Physical Workload and Ergonomic Factors Associated with Prevalence of Back and Neck Pain in Urban Transit Operators." Spine 22, no. 18 (1997): 2117-26.

Krause, N., D.R. Ragland, B.A. Greiner, S.L. Syme, and J.M. Fisher. "Psychological Job Factors Associated with Back and Neck Pain in Public Transit Operators." Scandinavian Journal of Work, Environment and Health 23, no. 3 (1997): 179-86. http://www.sjweh.fi/show_abstract.php?abstract_id=196.

Krause, N., R. Rugulier, D.R. Ragland, and S.L. Syme. "Physical Workload, Ergonomic Problems, and Incidence of Low Back Injury: A 7.5-Year Prospective Study of San Francisco Transit Operators." American Journal of Industrial Medicine 46, no. 6 (2004): 570-85. doi:10.1002/ajim.20094.

Kristiansen, T.K., J.P. Ryaby, J. McCabe, J.J. Frey, and L.R. Roe. "Accelerated Healing of Distal Radial Fractures with the Use of Specific Low-Intensity Ultrasound. A Multicenter, Prospective, Randomized, Double-Blind, Placebo-Controlled Study." Journal of Bone and Joint Surgery, American Volume 79, no. 7 (1997): 961-73. http://jbjs.org/article.aspx?articleid=23646.

Leung, K.S., W.S. Lee, H.F. Tsui, P.P. Liu, and W.H. Cheung. "Complex Tibial Fracture Outcomes Following Treatment with Low-Intensity Pulsed Ultrasound." Ultrasound in Medicine and Biology 30, no. 3 (2004): 389-95. http://www.umbjournal.org/article/S0301-5629(03)01199-2/abstract.

Linston, S.J. "A Review of Psychological Risk Factors in Back and Neck Pain." Spine 25, no. 9 (2000): 1148-56.

Malizos, K.N., M.E. Hantes, V. Protopappas, and A. Papachristos. "Low-Intensity Pulsed Ultrasound for Bone Healing: An Overview." Supplement,

Injury 37, no. S1 (2006): S56-62. doi:10.1016/j.injury.2006.02.037.

Marion, D.W., L.E. Penrod, S.F. Kelsey, W.D. Obrist, P.M. Kochanek, A.M. Palmer, and S.R. Wisniewski. "Treatment of Traumatic Brain Injury with Moderate Hypothermia." New England Journal of Medicine 336, no. 8 (1997): 540-46. http://www.nejm.org/doi/full/10.1056/NEJM199702203360803.

Mayr, E., M.M. Rudzki, M. Rudzki, B. Borchardt, H. Hausser, and A. Ruter. "Does Low Intensity, Pulsed Ultrasound Speed Healing of Scaphoid Fractures?" Handchirurgie, Mikrochirurgie, plastische Chirurgie: Organ der Deutschsprachigen 32 (2000): 115-22. https://www.thieme-connect.com/DOI/DOI?10.1055/s-2000-19253.

McCrory, P. "New Treatments for Concussion: The Next Millennium Beckons." Clinical Journal of Sport Medicine 11, no. 3 (2001): 190-93. http://journals.lww.com/cjsportsmed/pages/articleviewer.aspx?year=2001&issue=07000&article=00010&type=abstract.

McGarry, L.J., Thompson, D., Millham, F.H., Cowell, L., Snyder, P.J... Weinstein, M.C. "Outcomes and Costs of Acute Treatment of Traumatic Brain Injury." Journal of Trauma 53, no. 6 (2002): 1152-59. http://journals.lww.com/jtrauma/pages/articleviewer.aspx?year=2002&issue=12000&article=00020&type=abstract.

McGuirk, B., W. King, J. Govind, J. Lowry, and N. Bogduk. "Safety, Efficacy, and Cost Effectiveness of Evidence-Based Guidelines for the Management of Acute Low Back Pain in Primary Care." Spine 26, no. 23 (2001): 2615-22.

McIntyre, L.A., D.A. Fergusson, P.C. Hebert, D. Moher, and J.S. Hutchison. "Prolonged Therapeutic Hypothermia after Traumatic Brain Injury in Adults: A Systematic Review." Journal of the American Medical Association 289, no. 22 (2003): 2992-99. doi:10.1001/jama.289.22.2992.

Naravan, R.K. "Hypothermia for Traumatic Brain Injury—A Good Idea Proved Ineffective." New England Journal of Medicine 344, no. 8 (2001): 602-03. http://www.nejm.org/doi/full/10.1056/NEJM200102223440810.

National Committee for Quality Assurance. "Back Pain Recognition Program." BPRP Standards and Guidelines. http://www.ncqa.org/Programs/Recognition/BackPainRecognitionProgramBPRP.aspx.

North American Spine Society. Training Recommendations for New Technology. La Grange, IL: North American Spine Society, 2005. https://www.spine.org/Documents/general_new_techrecs.pdf.

North American Spine Society. North American Spine Society Phase III Clinical Guidelines for Multidisciplinary Spine Care Specialists. LaGrange, IL: North American Spine Society, 2000.

Ottawa Panel. "Ottawa Panel Evidence-Based Clinical Practice Guidelines for Therapeutic Exercises and Manual Therapy in the Management of Osteoarthritis." Physical Therapy 85, no. 9 (2005): 907-71. http://ptjournal.apta.org/content/85/9/907.long.

Peterson, C. "The Use of Electrical Stimulation and Taping to Address Shoulder

Subluxation for a Patient with Central Cord Syndrome." Physical Therapy 84, no. 7 (2004): 634-43. http://ptjournal.apta.org/content/84/7/634.long.

Philadelphia Panel. "Evidence-Based Clinical Practice Guidelines on Selected Rehabilitation Interventions: Overview and Methodology." Physical Therapy 81, no. 10 (2001): 1629-40. http://ptjournal.apta.org/content/81/10/1629.full.pdf+html.

Philadelphia Panel. "Evidence-Based Clinical Practice Guidelines on Selected Rehabilitation Interventions for Low Back Pain." Physical Therapy 81, no. 10 (2001): 1641-74. http://ptjournal.apta.org/content/81/10/1641.long.

Philadelphia Panel. "Evidence-Based Clinical Practice Guidelines on Selected Rehabilitation Interventions for Shoulder Pain." Physical Therapy 81, no. 10 (2001): 1719-30. http://ptjournal.apta.org/content/81/10/1719.long.

Philadelphia Panel. "Evidence-Based Clinical Practice Guidelines on Selected Rehabilitation Interventions for Knee Pain." Physical Therapy 81, no. 10 (2001): 1675-1700. http://ptjournal.apta.org/content/81/10/1675.long.

Quebec Task Force on Spinal Disorders. "Scientific Approach to the Assessment and Management of Activity-Related Spinal Disorders. A Monograph for Clinicians." Supplement, Spine 12, no. 1 7 (September 1987): S1-59.

Rand, S.E., C. Goerlich, K. Marchand, and N. Jablecki. "The Physical Therapy Prescription." American Family Physician 76, no. 11 (2007): 1661-66. http://www.aafp.org/afp/2007/1201/p1661.html.

Ricci, J.A., W.F. Stewart, E. Chee, C. Leotta, K. Foley, and M.C. Hochberg. "Back Pain Exacerbations and Lost Productive Time Costs in United States Workers." Spine 31, no. 26 (2006): 3052-60.

Robertson, V.J., and K.G. Baker. "A Review of Therapeutic Ultrasound: Effectiveness Studies." Physical Therapy 81, no. 7 (2001): 1339-40. http://ptjournal.apta.org/.

Roland, M., and J. Fairbank. "The Roland Disability Questionnaire." In The Back Pain Revolution, edited by Roland Waddell, 40. London: Churchill Livingstone, 2000.

Rothman, K.J. "Epidemiologic Methods in Clinical Trials." Supplement, Cancer 39, no. S4 (1977): 1771-75.

Rubin, C., M. Bolander, J.P. Ryaby, and M. Hadjiargyrou. The Use of Low-Intensity Ultrasound to Accelerate the Healing of Fractures." The Journal of Bone and Joint Surgery, American Volume 83-A, no. 2 (2001): 259-70. http://jbjs.org/article.aspx?articleid=24852.

Rutjes, A.W., E. Nuesch, R. Sterchi, and P. Juni. "Therapeutic Ultrasound for Osteoarthritis of the Knee or Hip." Cochrane Database System Review 20, no. 1 (2010). doi:10.1002/14651858.CD003132.pub2.

Sackett, D.L., and R.B. Haynes. "The Architecture of Diagnostic Research." BMJ 324, no. 7336 (2002): 539-41. http://www.ncbi.nlm.nih.gov/pmc/articles/PMC1122451/.

Santamato, A., Solfrizzi, V., Panza, F., Tondi, G., Frisardi, V., Leggin, B.G...Fiore, P. "Short-Term Effects of High-Intensity Laser Therapy versus Ultrasound Therapy in the Treatment of People with Subacromial Impingement Syndrome: A Randomized Clinical Trial." Physical Therapy 89, no. 7 (2009): 643-52. doi:10.2522/ptj.20080139.

Scalzitti, D.A. "Evidence-Based Guidelines: Application to Clinical Practice." Physical Therapy 81, no. 10 (2001): 1622-28. http://ptjournal.apta.org/content/81/10/1622.full?sid=c5922cf4-229a-4568-81c5-521316f0bc7d.

Sherry, E., P. Kitchener, and R. Smart. "A Prospective Randomized Controlled Study of VAX-D and TENS for the Treatment of Chronic Low Back Pain." Neurological Research 23, no. 7 (2001): 780-85.

Speed, C. "Low Back Pain." BMJ 328, no. 7448 (2004): 1119-21. http://www.ncbi.nlm.nih.gov/pubmed/15130982.

Speed, C.A. "Therapeutic Ultrasound in Soft Tissue Lesions." Rheumatology 40, no. 12 (2001): 1331-36. doi:10.1093/rheumatology/40.12.1331.

State of Colorado. "Special Instructions for Rule 17 Medical Treatment Guidelines Exhibits 1-10." Colorado Treatment Guidelines Denver: State of Colorado, 2006. http://www.colorado.gov/cs/Satellite/CDLE-WorkComp/CDLE/1248095315991.

Straub, S.J., L.D. Johns, and S.M. Howard. "Variability in Effective Radiating Area at 1 Mhz Affects Ultrasound Treatment Intensity." Physical Therapy 88, no. 1 (2008): 50-57. http://ptjournal.apta.org/content/88/1/50.long.

Van Tulder, M., Becker, A., Bekkering, T., Breen A, del Real, M.T., Hutchinson, A...Laerum, E. "Chapter 3: European Guidelines for the Management of Acute Nonspecific Low Back Pain in Primary Care." Supplement, European Spine Journal 15, no. S2 (2006): S169-91. http://link.springer.com/article/10.1007%2Fs00586-006-1071-2.

Van Tulder, M., A. Furlan, C. Bombardier, and L. Bouter. "Updated Method Guidelines for Systematic Reviews in the Cochrane Collaboration Back Review Group." Spine 28, no. 12 (2003): 1290-99. http://www.ncbi.nlm.nih.gov/pubmed/12811274.

Waddell, G., and A.K. Burton. "Occupational Health Guidelines for the Management of Low Back Pain at Work. Evidence Review and Recommendations." Occupational Medicine 51, no. 2 (2001): 124-35. http://occmed.oxfordjournals.org/content/51/2/124.long.

Warden, S.J., R.K. Fuchs, C.K. Kessler, K.G. Avin, R.E. Cardinal, and R.L. Stewart. "Ultrasound Produced by a Conventional Therapeutic Ultrasound Unit Accelerates Fracture Repair." Physical Therapy 86, no. 8 (2006): 1118-27. http://ptjournal.apta.org/content/86/8/1118.long.

Wieder, D.L. "Treatment of Traumatic Myositis Ossificans with Ascetic Acid Iontophoresis." Physical Therapy 72, no. 2 (1992): 133-37.

Wong, R.A., B. Schumann, R. Townsend, and C.A. Phelps. "A Survey of Therapeutic Ultrasound Use by Physical Therapists Who Are Orthopaedic Certified Specialists." Physical Therapy 87, no. 8 (2007): 986-94. doi:10.2522/ptj.20050392.

Work Loss Data Institute. Low Back—Lumbar & Thoracic (Acute & Chronic).

Encinitas, CA: Work Loss Data Institute, 2011. http://guideline.gov/content. aspx?id=33184.

Wupperman, R., R. Davis, and W.T. Obremskey. "Level of Evidence in Spine Compared to Other Orthopedic Journals." Spine 32, no. 3 (2007): 338-93. http://www.ncbi.nlm.nih.gov/pubmed/17268275.

Examination

Upon meeting the Satisfactory Completion Statement, you may receive a certificate of completion at the end of this course.

Contact ceu@rehabsurge.com to find out if this distance learning course is an approved course from your board. Save your course outline and contact your own board or organization for specific filing requirements.

In order to obtain continuing education hours, you must have read the book, have completed the exam and survey. Please include a $30.00 exam fee for your exam. Mail the exam answer sheet and survey sheet to:

Rehabsurge, Inc.

PO Box 287

Baldwin, NY 11510

Allow 2–4 weeks to receive your certificate.

You can also take the exam online at www.rehabsurge.com. Register and pay the exam fee of $30.00. After you passed the exam with a score of 70%, you will be able to print your certificate immediately. See rehabsurge.com for more details.

Exam Questions

1. This type of clinical practice guideline include a measure of the effectiveness of evidence based recommendations within the guideline to determine whether the recommendation improved the quality of care.
   a. expert-based
   b. preference-based
   c. outcome-based
   c. patient based

2. This type of modality uses electric current deliver ionically charged substances through the skin to deeper tissues.
   a. Ultrasound
   b. Phonophoresis
   c. Iontophoresis
   d. Low level laser therapy

3. This modality generates an action potential in nerve tissue, causing a muscle contraction or altering sensory input.
   a. Electrical stimulation
   b. Infrared
   c. Paraffin wax bath
   d. Vertebral decompression

4. The acoustic energy generated from ultrasound is produced from a piezoelectric crystal within a transducer, which emits high-frequency acoustic pressure waves that are transmitted through body tissues by molecular vibrations and collisions. These pressure waves are equal to:
   a. 1-12 MHz
   b. 15-20 Mhz
   c. 21-30 Mhz
   d. 10-25 Mhz

5. Which bone is the most commonly fractured long bone and accounts for 35-65% of all nonunions?
   a. clavicle
   b. femur
   c. radius
   d. tibia

6. Which modality has been used in the treatment of nonunions, with the premise that these high energy waves cause microfracture of the bone trabeculae and through this tissue damage encourage the reparative process leading to fracture union?
a. transcutaneous electrical nerve stimulation
b. functional electrical stimulation
c. orthotripsy
d. low level laser therapy

7. Which stage of fracture healing commences with the disruption of blood vessels from the injury and the formation of a hematoma?
a. inflammatory
b. reparative
c. remodeling
d. scar formation

8. The definition of a delayed union is generally thought to be healing not completed by __ months.
a. 1 month
b. 2 months
c. 3 months
d. 6 months

9. The formation of tiny gas bubbles in the tissues as the result of ultrasound vibration is called:
a. piezoelectric effect
b. phonophoresis
c. shock wave
d. cavitation

10. Which condition is an age-related disease of the joints characterized by focal areas of loss of articular cartilage in synovial joints, accompanied by subchondral bone changes, osteophyte formation at the joint margins, thickening of the joint capsule and mild synovitis?
a. Osteoarthritis
b. Rheumatoid arthritis
c. Psoriatic arthritis
d. Gouty arthritis

11. Which frequency of adjunctive noncontact ultrasound appears to improve healing in wounds that fail to heal with conventional wound care alone?
    a. 10 kHz
    b. 20 kHz
    c. 30 kHz
    d. 40 kHz

12. What condition is characterized by heterotopic ossification (calcification) of muscle? Calcification usually appears within 2 to 3 weeks.
    a. Myositis ossificans
    b. Bursitis
    c. Calcific tendinitis
    d. Impingement

13. Nausea has been reported with prolonged use of this modality.
    a. Mechanical traction
    b. Electrical stimulation
    c. Low level laser therapy
    d. Ultrasound

14. Which substance prevents the proliferation of prostaglandin E?
    a. cytomchrome oxidase
    b. superoxide dismutase
    c. cytokine
    d. endorphin

15. Intermittent or continuous force applied along the long axis of the spine, in an attempt to elongate the spine, or the act of pulling or stretching muscle or joints is performed by this modality.
    a. Traction
    b. Electrical stimulation
    c. Low level laser therapy
    d. Ultrasound

16. The VAX-D table asserts its effect through decompression of the intervertebral disc and has reduced intradiscal pressures to a negative ___ mm Hg.
a. 100
b. 150
c. 200
d. 250

17. Grade B recommendation is defined by:
a. good evidence to include intervention
b. fair evidence to include intervention
c. poor evidence to include or exclude intervention
d. insufficient data

18. A patient is said to suffer from rheumatoid arthritis if he/she satisfies at least 4 of the following 7 American Rheumatism Association criteria. These include:
a. morning stiffness;
b. arthritis of 3 or more joints
c. arthritis of the hand joints;
d. symmetric involvement of joints

19. Therapeutic ultrasound in rheumatoid arthritis of the hand was included in the placebo controlled randomized trial. Continuous wave ultrasound was applied in water to the dorsal and palmar aspects of the hand at 0.5 W/cm^2. What was the prescribed frequency?
a. 10 minutes on alternative days for 3 weeks for a total of 10 sessions
b. 10 minutes on alternative days for 3 weeks for a total of 20 sessions
c. 8 minutes on alternative days for 3 weeks for a total of 10 sessions
d. 8 minutes on alternative days for 3 weeks for a total of 20 sessions

20. This condition is a rheumatologic disorder that requires the concurrent existence of chronic, widespread musculoskeletal pain and multiple sites of tenderness.
a. myofascial pain syndrome
b. fibromyalgia
c. scleroderma
d. rheumatoid arthritis

Answer sheet

Name:_____

Address:_____

Profession:_____

License Number:_____

Date:_____

E-mail Address (optional):_____

Exam:

1.	a	b	c	d
2.	a	b	c	d
3.	a	b	c	d
4.	a	b	c	d
5.	a	b	c	d
6.	a	b	c	d
7.	a	b	c	d
8.	a	b	c	d
9.	a	b	c	d
10.	a	b	c	d
11.	a	b	c	d
12.	a	b	c	d
13.	a	b	c	d
14.	a	b	c	d
15.	a	b	c	d
16.	a	b	c	d
17.	a	b	c	d
18.	a	b	c	d
19.	a	b	c	d
20.	a	b	c	d

Please mail $30.00 and completed form to:

CEU certificate request
Rehabsurge, Inc.
PO Box 287
Baldwin, NY 11510.
Contact Us at:
Phone: +1 (516) 515-1267
Email: ceu@rehabsurge.com

Alternatively, you can take the exam online at **www.rehabsurge.com**
You will receive your certificate instantly.

It is the learner's responsibility to comply with all state and national regulatory board's rules and regulations. This includes but is not limited to:
•verifying and complying with applicable continuing education requirements;
•verifying and complying with all applicable standards of practice;
•verifying and complying with all licensure requirements;
•any other rules or laws identified in the learners state or regulatory board that is not mentioned here.
It is the learner's responsibility to complete ALL coursework in order to receive credit. This includes but is not limited to:
•Reading all course materials fully;
•Completing all course activities to meet the criteria set forth by the instructor;
•Completing and passing all applicable tests and quizzes. All learner's MUST take a comprehensive online exam where they MUST get at least 70%. Getting 70% is a requirement to pass.

IMPORTANT. Rehabsurge reserves the right to deny continuing education credits or withdraw credits issued at any time if: Coursework is found to be incomplete, It is determined that a user falsified, copied, and/or engaged in any flagrant attempt to manipulate, modify, or alter the coursework just to receive credit; and/or It is determined that the coursework was not completed by the user.

If any of the conditions above are determined, Rehabsurge reserves the right to notify any applicable state and national boards along with supporting documentation.

Program Evaluation Form

Rehabsurge, Inc. works to develop new programs based on your comments and suggestions, making your feedback on the program very important to us. We would appreciate you taking a few moments to evaluate this program.

Course Start Date:_____   Course End Date: _____

Course Start Time:_____   Course End Time:_____

Identity Verification: Name:_____

Profession:_____ License Number:_____State: _____

Please initial to indicate that you are the individual who read the book and completed the test.
Initial here:_____

May we use your comments and suggestions in upcoming marketing materials.   Yes   No

Would you take another seminar from Rehabsurge, Inc.?   Yes   No

The educational level required to read the book is: Beginner Intermediate   Advanced

The course is:	(5-Yes/Excellent)			(1- No/Poor)	
Relevant to my profession	5	4	3	2	1
Valuable to my profession	5	4	3	2	1
Content matched stated objectives	5	4	3	2	1
Complete coverage of materials	5	4	3	2	1
Teaching ability	5	4	3	2	1
Organization of material	5	4	3	2	1
Effective	5	4	3	2	1

Please rate the objectives. After reading the material, how well do you feel you are able to meet:

Objective 1	5	4	3	2	1
Objective 2	5	4	3	2	1
Objective 3	5	4	3	2	1
Objective 4	5	4	3	2	1
Objective 5	5	4	3	2	1

What was the most beneficial part of the program? What was the least beneficial part of the program?
_____
_____
_____
_____

What would you like to see added to the program? In what ways might we make this program experience better for you?_____
_____
_____
_____
_____

If you have any general comments on this topic or program please explain.
_____
_____
_____
_____

Please tell us what other programs or topics might interest you?
_____
_____
_____
_____

Thank you for participating and taking the time to join us today!

Made in the USA
San Bernardino, CA
08 January 2014